Infection and Imm

KING ALFRED'S
WINCHESTER

Infection and Immunity

**D.H. Davies, M.A. Halablab, J. Clarke,
F.E.G. Cox and T.W.K. Young**

School of Health and Life Sciences
King's College, London

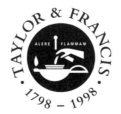

TAYLOR & FRANCIS

ALERE FLAMMAM

· 1798 – 1998 ·

UK   Taylor & Francis Ltd, 1 Gunpowder Square, London, EC4A 3DE
USA Taylor & Francis Inc., 1900 Frost Road, Suite 101, Bristol, PA 19007

British Library Cataloguing in Publication Data

A catalogue record for this book is available from the British Library.
ISBN 0-7484-0788-X (paper)

Library of Congress Cataloguing-in-Publication Data are available

Cover design by Jim Wilkie
Typeset in Melior 10/12.5pt by Graphicraft Ltd, Hong Kong
Printed and bound by T.J. International Ltd, Padstow, Cornwall
Cover printed by Flexiprint, Lancing, West Sussex

Contents

General Preface to the Series

The curriculum for higher education now presents most degree programmes as a collection of discrete packages or modules. The modules stand alone but, as a set, comprise a general programme of study. Usually around half of the modules taken by the undergraduate are compulsory and count as a core curriculum for the final degree. The arrangement has the advantage of flexibility. The range of options over and above the core curriculum allows the student to choose the best programme for his or her future.

Usually, the subject of the core curriculum, for example biochemistry, has a general textbook that covers the material at length. Smaller specialist volumes deal in depth with particular topics, for example photosynthesis or muscle contraction. The optional subjects in a modular system, however, are too many for the student to buy the general textbook for each and the small in-depth titles generally do not cover sufficient material. The new series *Modules in Life Sciences* provides a selection of texts which can be used at the undergraduate level for subjects optional to the main programme of study. Each volume aims to cover the material at a depth suitable to a particular year of undergraduate study with an amount appropriate to a module, usually around one-quarter of the undergraduate year. The life sciences was chosen as the general subject area since it is here, more than most, that individual topics proliferate. For example, a student of biochemistry may take optional modules in physiology, microbiology, medical pathology and even mathematics.

Suggestions for new modules and comments on the present volume will always be welcomed and should be addressed to the series editor.

John Wrigglesworth, Series Editor
King's College, London

Preface

This book was born out of the need for an inexpensive text to accompany a very popular 3rd year course, also entitled 'Infection & Immunity', that we offer to students in the Division of Life Sciences at King's College. In this course we use a few specific examples from the world of human pathogens – viruses, bacteria, fungi, protozoa and helminths – to illustrate the relationship between pathogen and human host; specifically, the ways in which specialized pathogens have become adapted to their human host, the means by which the immune system normally protects against such pathogens, and the means by which some pathogens evade immunity and cause disease. As one referee put it: a disease-based approach to immunology. No doubt there are similar courses in other universities with similar objectives. However, one major problem associated with drawing from such a diverse collection of microorganisms is that no single textbook can provide the necessary background. No student can be expected to buy textbooks in immunology, virology, microbiology, mycology and parasitology for a single course! We do not claim that this book is comprehensive – that would defeat its purpose. Instead this book will provide a companion to your 'Infection & Immunity' course and through references provided at the end of each chapter, will direct you to further reading should you wish to delve deeper into a particular subject. We apologize to our colleagues who feel we have omitted something important – that is inevitable in a book of this nature. Also, any mistakes you may find are entirely our own fault. In short, the authors welcome any constructive criticisms or comments for future editions of this book.

Huw Davies, Mahmoud Halablab, John Clarke,
Frank Cox, Tom Young
London, March 1998

1 The Immune System

In this chapter we will examine the immune system. It will not be possible to provide a detailed account of immunology in a single chapter, and it will help if the reader has at least some background in the subject. Instead, this chapter will emphasize those aspects of immunology that will be important for understanding the significance of material to follow. Here we will focus on two broad areas. First, the different **effector mechanisms** of the immune system that neutralize and kill invading microorganisms. Secondly, we will examine T-cell function and focus mainly on **antigen processing** and the functions of T_H1 and T_H2 cells. Several excellent reviews are listed at the end of this chapter if further information is required.

1.1 Epithelium is the first line of defence

Humans are host to many diverse microorganisms which coexist in, or on, our bodies at some stage during their life cycle. Many are a normal component of our microbial flora which colonize the external epithelial surfaces or the epithelial linings of the respiratory, alimentary or genital tracts. For the most part, the relationship is of little consequence to us and such microorganisms are termed **commensal**. However, damage to the epithelium may allow otherwise harmless commensal microorganisms to breach the protective epithelium, enter the tissues or be disseminated by the circulatory system. Invasion by microbes may also be accompanied by their multiplication (**infection**), in which case disease – a state of illness or a reduced competence to function normally – often occurs. The causes of disease are numerous but are often the result of damage to the cells or tissues of the body caused by multiplication of the microbes, or by the release of toxic metabolic by-products or components found in their cell walls. Any microorganism that causes disease is called a **pathogen**.

The integrity of the epithelium is therefore vital to block the entry of microbes. Epithelial cells are joined by tight junctions and epithelium normally represents an impenetrable barrier to most microorganisms. This physical barrier is supplemented by chemicals with a variety of microbicidal

Table 1.1   Epithelial barriers to microbial infection

Physical	Epithelial cells joined by tight junctions Exfoliation of surface cells Mucus flow by ciliated epithelia (respiratory tract)

Chemical	Enzymes: lysozyme (tears, saliva, sweat)
	               pepsin (stomach)
	Low pH: fatty acids/amino acids (skin)
	               gastric acids (stomach)
	Antimicrobial: transferrin (mucus)

Microbial	Normal flora (gut)

properties (Table 1.1). These include **lysozyme** and **transferrin**. Lysozyme cleaves peptidoglycan in microbial cell walls and is particularly effective against Gram-positive bacteria. Transferrin inhibits microbial growth by sequestering essential iron. The physical barrier of epithelium is also helped by resident commensal microbes that compete with potentially pathogenic microbes for nutrients and available space for attachment. If a microbe was to breach the epithelium it would multiply and soon overwhelm the host unless rapidly mobilizable defence reactions were present. In addition to the opportunistic microorganisms that gain entry through breaches in the epithelium, there are many other species of microorganism that have become specialists at actively invading the body and colonizing a particular anatomical niche, such as a particular cell type or organ. Such relationships have usually been accompanied by the evolution of a variety of strategies for evading the immune system. It is from these types of pathogens that we have learned much about the immune system, and which form the examples used in this book.

1.2   Pathogens that breach epithelium are eliminated by defence reactions

The defence reactions that are activated in response to damaged epithelium are:

- Blood clotting (coagulation). This is caused by the activation of the fibrinogen cascade that serves to seal haemorrhages and entrap and prevent the dispersal of any microorganisms that have gained entry.
- Inflammation. This can be triggered directly by microbes or by physical trauma alone, and causes increased blood flow and permeability of the capillaries in the region of the injury or infection. This allows cells and fluid to leave the capillaries and enter the site, resulting in the

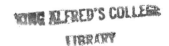

four classic symptoms of inflammation: swelling, redness, heat and pain. The function of inflammation is twofold: first, to allow cellular and humoral components of the immune system to infiltrate the site to assist in the removal of any invading microorganisms; secondly, to allow infiltrating cells to assist in the repair of any connective tissue damage.

- The immune system. The function of the immune system is to kill or neutralize the microorganisms and to retain a 'memory' of an exposure to a particular pathogen so that subsequent encounters elicit a much more rapid specific response.

Although outside the scope of this book, it should be mentioned here that immune responses triggered by microbes can lead to exacerbation of disease, or entirely new diseases, either as a result of chronic overstimulation by microbes, or by stimulation at an inappropriate time or place. These immune pathologies appear to be an unavoidable consequence of having such an effective immune system, and include the various hypersensitivities (such as allergies) and the auto-immune diseases (such as rheumatoid arthritis and auto-immune diabetes).

1.3 Innate and adaptive mechanisms together form the immune system

The first components encountered by microorganisms that penetrate epithelial barriers are the cells and molecules of the innate immune system (Table 1.2). Innate reactions include **phagocytosis** by macrophages, triggering of the alternative pathway of the **complement cascade**, and killing of infected cells by **natural killer (NK) cells**. Recognition is by preformed receptors able to recognize structures on a broad range on microbes. Moreover, the effector cells are numerous and their response is mobilized immediately the microbes gain entry. Most organisms that penetrate are recognized and destroyed within a few hours by the innate system.

Only if a few organisms breach this early line of innate defence is the adaptive response mobilized (Table 1.2). Adaptive immunity is mediated by **lymphocytes** which use specific antigen receptors. Only in the presence of essential costimulatory signals elicited by inflammation do lymphocytes respond to microbial antigens. Antigen receptors are produced during lymphocyte ontogeny by a process of gene rearrangement. This generates a repertoire of several billion different receptors which endows each of us with the

Table 1.2   Cells and molecules of innate and adaptive immunity

	Main functions
Innate	
Mast cells	Degranulate in response to tissue injury to release histamine and other substances that trigger inflammation (attracts phagocytes; allows phagocytes and fluid containing complement to enter from blood)
Eosinophils	Degranulate on surface of helminth worms coated with IgE antibody
Macrophages	Phagocytosis and killing of extracellular pathogens (recognition using own innate receptors or after opsonization by complement components or antibodies) Present antigen to T_H0 cells and promote their differentiation into T_H1 cells Become activated by T_H1 and NK cells to become more microbicidal and to promote inflammation
Neutrophils	Phagocytosis and killing of extracellular pathogens

Complement	Enzymatic cascade that generates many components in host defence, including:
	    opsonins (coat microbes for phagocytosis)
	    chemotactic factors for phagocytes
	    anaphylatoxins (trigger mast cell and basophil degranulation)
	    membrane attack complex (disrupts cell membranes)

Natural killer (NK) cells	Killing of infected cells (recognition by own innate receptor, or after coating of infected cell with antibody – a process called antibody-dependent cell-mediated cytotoxicity or ADCC) Activation of macrophages
Langerhans cells	Cutaneous antigen-presenting cells that capture antigen and migrate to draining secondary lymphoid tissue (to become interdigitating dendritic cells) where they activate naive antigen-specific T lymphocytes
Adaptive immunity	
CD4+ T lymphocytes	After activation by antigen (by peptide/class II MHC on dendritic cells) in secondary lymphoid tissue, differentiate into T_H1 or T_H2 cells

	T_H1 ('inflammatory' or DTH*) cells:
	    activate macrophages to become more microbicidal
	    induce B lymphocytes to produce opsonizing antibody
	    suppress differentiation of T_H2 cells

	T_H2 ('helper') cells:
	    induce B cells to produce antibody
	    suppress inflammation by inhibiting macrophage activation and differentiation of T_H1 cells

CD8+ T lymphocytes	After activation by antigen (by peptide/class I MHC) differentiate into cytotoxic T lymphocytes (T_C cells) and kill infected or tumour cells

Table 1.2 Cont'd

	Main functions
B lymphocytes	Capture antigen with surface Ig (IgD, IgM) which is then ingested and processed into peptides. Peptides presented at cell surface by class II MHC molecules to activated T_H2 cells; cytokines and costimulation from T_H2 cause B cells to differentiate into plasma cells that secrete Ig (antibodies)

	Antibodies have several functions in immunity to extracellular pathogens:
	  Neutralization and agglutination of microbes and toxins (most Ig, especially IgG, IgM)
	  Opsonization of microbes for phagocytosis (IgG1, IgG3)
	  activation of complement cascade by classic pathway (IgM, IgG)
	  Sensitization of mast cells and eosinophils in helminth immunity and allergy (IgE)
	  Secretion into fluids (mucus, tears, saliva) to mediate neutralization (IgA)

	Antibodies can also mediate killing of infected cells: ADCC by NK cells (Ig1, IgG3)

* DTH, delayed type hypersensitivity.

capacity to recognize any antigen that we may encounter during our lifetimes. Lymphocytes are normally in a state of metabolic quiescence and only become activated after encountering specific antigen to differentiate into effector cells. Lymphocytes comprise **B cells** and **T cells**. After activation, B cells differentiate into plasma cells which manufacture soluble antigen receptors called **antibodies**. T cells can be subclassified according to the expression of the coreceptors, CD4 and CD8. Cells bearing CD8 differentiate into **cytotoxic T lymphocytes** (T_C cells) whose function is to kill host cells that are infected by intracellular microbes such as viruses. In contrast, T cells bearing CD4 differentiate along different pathways that are defined by the particular cocktail of cytokines they secrete. At the opposite ends of this spectrum are T_H1 and T_H2 cells, which are instrumental in helping the development of cell-mediated and humoral immunity, respectively.

If the host has not been exposed to the antigen before, antigen-specific lymphocytes are rare in the repertoire and must undergo clonal expansion and differentiation into effector cells before the microorganisms can be removed. The adaptive system is therefore slow to respond (more than 4 days) to the primary exposure of a pathogen. However, unlike the innate system, an adaptive response leaves behind a pool of previously activated 'memory' lymphocytes and preformed antibodies that can act immediately upon a subsequent infection. This ensures that an individual becomes protected or immune to a particular pathogen (see reviews of memory by Ahmed and Grey, 1996; Sprent, 1997). This is also the phenomenon that is exploited by vaccination (discussed in Chapter 6).

At this point it is important to mention that the delay in mounting an adaptive response allows many pathogens to survive in their hosts by constantly changing their antigens (**antigenic variation**). This may occur randomly as the pathogen replicates, as is the case with many RNA viruses such as influenza (sections 3.2 and 3.3) and the human immunodeficiency virus (section 3.4), or by having several stages to their life cycle, as is the case with some protozoan parasites such as *Plasmodium* (section 4.4). Several species of bacteria and fungi also employ this as a means of escape. In each case the organism remains one step ahead of the developing adaptive response (see review by Deitsch *et al.*, 1997). Antigenic variation is also a major hurdle to be overcome in the design of vaccines against rapidly changing pathogens.

It is important to remember that the adaptive system has evolved over the older pre-existing innate system, and there is a strong interdependence between the two systems. There are numerous instances where the same effector mechanisms (such as macrophage activation, inflammation, and activation of the complement cascade) can be triggered by either innate or antigen receptors. Moreover, antigen receptors have no inherent capacity to discriminate self antigens from those of pathogens. The apparent ability of the immune system to discriminate between self and foreign is due in part to the inactivation or removal from the repertoire of potentially harmful autoreactive lymphocytes. This leads to a state of non-responsiveness to self antigens called **tolerance** and leaves a residual repertoire that retains lymphocytes specific for non-self or foreign antigen (reviewed by Goodnow, 1996; Mondino *et al.*, 1996). However, foreign antigen is, in itself, insufficient to trigger an adaptive response; this requires stimulatory cytokines and other mediators that are first generated by inflammation and by the cells and molecules of the innate immune system (see reviews by Fearon and Locksley, 1996; Mondino *et al.*, 1996).

1.4   Responses to extracellular pathogens

The type of effector mechanism elicited by the innate and adaptive immune systems is largely determined by whether

Table 1.3 Immunity to extracellular and intracellular pathogens

Type of pathogen	Examples	Effector cells or mechanism
Extracellular	Viruses, bacteria, protozoa, fungi, helminth worms	Antibodies, complement, phagocytes, mast cells/eosinophils (worms)
Intracellular, cytosolic	Viruses Some bacteria: *Listeria* spp. *Chlamydia*	NK cells, ADCC, T_C lymphocytes
Intracellular, endosomal	Bacteria: *Mycobacterium tuberculosis* *Mycobacterium leprae* *Salmonella typhimurium* *Legionella pneumophila* *Listeria* spp. Protozoa: *Leishmania* spp. *Plasmodium* spp. *Trypanosoma* spp. *Toxoplasma gondii*	Macrophages activated by T_H1 cells and NK cells

the microbe inhabits an intracellular or extracellular environment in the body (Table 1.3). Extracellular pathogens include all fungi and helminth worms (flukes, tapeworms and nematodes), and the majority of bacteria. Also included in this category are the normally intracellular pathogens such as viruses, some species of bacteria and protozoan parasites, in the stage of their life cycle prior to invading a host cell.

1.4.1 *Complement*

Complement is an innate effector mechanism consisting of an enzymatic cascade of over 30 preformed serum and cell-surface components (see reviews by Frank and Freis, 1991; Kinoshita, 1991). The cascade can be triggered directly by the cell walls of microorganisms (the **alternative pathway**), or indirectly by the binding of antibodies to the microbial surface (the **classical pathway**). These pathways are summarized in Figure 1.1. The classical pathway can also be triggered by lectins that bind to sugar residues on the cell walls of pathogens (reviewed by Matsushita, 1996). At each stage, inactive substrates are cleaved to produce two or more by-products with biological properties. Some possess enzymatic activity of their own and activate the downstream components, while others have antimicrobial or proinflammatory properties. Although these two pathways use different

Figure 1.1

Overview of the alternative and classical pathways of complement activation.

In the alternative pathway, C3 in plasma undergoes spontaneous cleavage into C3a and C3b. C3b has a labile thioester bond that will covalently bond to microorganisms and cell membranes nearby or react harmlessly with water. Once bound to a cell surface, C3b binds factor B which is cleaved into Ba and Bb by a protease, factor D. C3bBb is a C3 convertase that cleaves more C3 causing a positive feedback amplification and deposition of C3b on the cell surface. On healthy cells in the body, different complement control proteins (CR1, DAF, factor H and MCP) bind and displace Bb (see Liszewski *et al.*, 1996). Bb is then cleaved by factor I to give iC3b (inactive C3b). However, on microbial surfaces that lack these control proteins, C3bBb is stabilized by factor P leading to the deposition of more C3b on the pathogen. In the classical pathway the cascade is triggered by the binding of antibody to the pathogen surface. Plasma C1, the first component in this pathway, is a complex of three different types of subunits, C1q, C1r and C1s. C1q binds to the Fc regions of bound IgM or IgG which cleaves and activates the C1s subunits. Activated C1s then cleaves plasma C4 into C4a and C4b. C4b then binds to plasma C2 which becomes cleaved by C1s to produce C2a and C2b. The C4a and C2b components diffuse away, whereas the membrane-bound C4b2a complex is the C3 convertase of the classical pathway and results in the deposition of C3a on the pathogen. Several of the cleavage by-products generated by these two pathways have important proinflammatory and antimicrobial activities (see Table 1.4). Thereafter the two pathways converge on the common lytic pathway (components C5 to C9) culminating in the formation of the membrane attack complex (Figure 1.2).

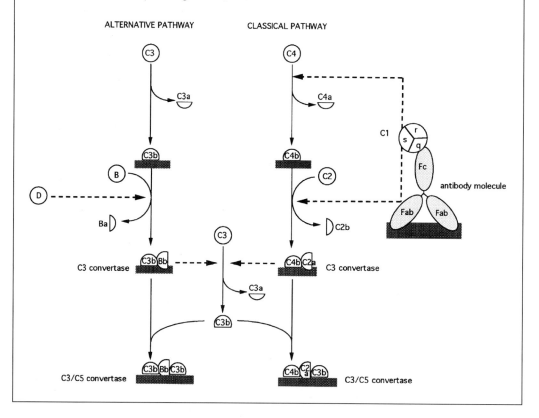

Table 1.4 Products generated by the complement cascade that have important antimicrobial properties

Product	Property	Notes
C2a	Vasoactive	Causes vasodilation and increased vascular permeability
C3a	Anaphylatoxic	Causes mast cells and basophils to release vasoactive agents such as histamine
	Chemotactic	Attracts phagocytes
C3b	Opsonic	Bound by CR1* (CD35) on phagocytes CR1 also involved with regulatory factor I in degrading C3b
	Antigen trapping	CR1 receptor on follicular dendritic cells
iC3b	Opsonic	Bound by integrins CR3 (CD11b/CD18) and CR4 (CD11c/CD18) on phagocytes and NK cells
C4a	Anaphylatoxic	Causes mast cells and basophils to release vasoactive agents such as histamine
C4b	Opsonic	Bound by CR1 (CD35) on phagocytes CR1 also involved with regulatory factor I in degrading C4b
C5a	Anaphylatoxic	Causes mast cells and basophils to release vasoactive agents such as histamine
	Haemostatic	Causes platelet aggregation
	Chemotactic	Attracts phagocytes Increases expression of complement receptors (CR3 and CR4) on neutrophils

* CR, complement receptor.

components, several components from one pathway have homologues in the other suggesting they have evolved from common ancestral genes. Cells in the body are protected from complement by a system of control proteins (see Liszewski *et al.*, 1996). These are cell-surface and serum inhibitors that are absent from the surfaces of microorganisms.

Table 1.4 lists the important cleavage products generated by the two pathways that assist in the removal of micro-organisms. Of importance here are **chemotactic factors** and **opsonins**. Chemotactic factors guide phagocytes (macrophages and neutrophils) toward the source of the factor in the direction of increasing concentration (**chemotaxis**), thereby enabling phagocytes to locate and ingest the microorganisms. Opsonins are substances that bind to the microbial surface and enable phagocytes that bear receptors for opsonins to bind and ingest the microbes more efficiently.

Thereafter, both pathways converge on a common **lytic pathway** that culminates in the assembly of the **membrane attack complex** (MAC), represented in Figure 1.2. The MAC forms pores in cell membranes and may be important for damaging pathogens surrounded by accessible lipid

Figure 1.2
Formation of the membrane attack complex.
C3b binds to the C3 convertase produced by either pathway
forming a C5 convertase that cleaves C5 into C5b, releasing
C5a. C6, C7 and C8 assemble sequentially in the membrane
while multiple C9 subunits polymerize forming a pore in the
membrane.

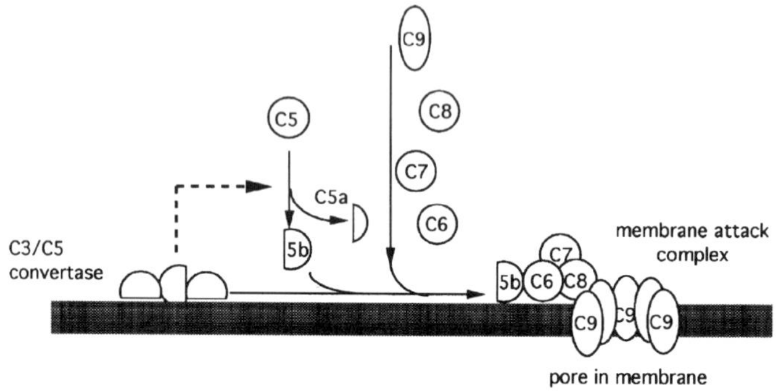

membranes such as enveloped viruses. However, its importance seems to be limited, and the opsonic, chemotactic and
proinflammatory components of the earlier stages appear
more important in host defence.

1.4.2　*Phagocytosis and triggering of inflammation*

The major phagocytes in the body are **tissue macrophages**
and **neutrophils**. Macrophages are amoeboid cells found
moving throughout the connective tissues ingesting extracellular debris and effete cells. These cells originate continu-
ously from blood-borne monocytes that enter the tissues by
migrating through blood capillaries. Macrophages are also
attracted by chemotactic factors released by mast cells that
degranulate in response to tissue injury. The macrophages
then participate in ingesting microorganisms that may have
gained entry. In the process, macrophages become stimulated
and release cytokines, **interleukin-1 (IL-1), IL-6** and **tumour
necrosis factor-α (TNF-α)**, that have overlapping inflammatory properties. Local effects include activation of vascular
endothelium. This increases vascular permeability to allow
complement, and later antibodies, to enter the site of infection, and to increase the drainage of fluid and cells to lymph
nodes. IL-1 and TNF-α also increase expression of adhesion
molecules on vascular endothelium to make it more adhes-

ive for neutrophils and, later, activated T lymphocytes. The systemic effects of these cytokines are to act on the hypothalamus to induce fever to retard the growth of microorganisms, and induce production of **acute-phase proteins** by liver hepatocytes (see below). During phagocytosis, macrophages also release **IL-8**, which is a chemotactic cytokine (chemokine) for neutrophils, and complement proteins which, as we have seen, assist in the removal of microbes and enhance inflammation.

Neutrophils are normally found in the blood but are attracted during the acute (early) stage of inflammation by the cytokines produced by the macrophages. In the later stages of inflammation, monocytes also infiltrate sites of inflammation wherein they can differentiate into more tissue macrophages.

Many pathogens can be recognized directly by phagocytes by virtue of their possession of innate receptors for microbial cell-wall components, such as complement receptor 3 (CR3), and the mannose receptor, which both bind to structures on the surface of many microorganisms directly (reviewed by Ofek *et al.*, 1995). However, this is a relatively inefficient means of binding to microorganisms. A more efficient means of uptake is if the microbe is first opsonized, which increases the avidity of the interaction between the opsonized microbe and the phagocyte bearing appropriate opsonin receptors. There are three basic categories of opsonin, each generated at different stages during an immune response.

- Opsonins produced by activation of the complement cascade (see Table 1.4). Because the components of the cascade are preformed, complement-derived opsonins are the first to appear.
- Acute-phase proteins produced by the liver in response to the inflammatory cytokines (IL-1, IL-6 and TNF-α). These include **C-reactive protein** which binds to microbial lipopolysaccharide (LPS), and **mannose-binding protein** which is a lectin that binds to mannose residues in bacterial cell walls. Both are opsonins and are able to trigger the complement cascade (see Turner, 1996).
- Antibodies. Several subclasses of antibodies are opsonic and are bound by Fc receptors on phagocytes. Not all microbes can be recognized by the opsonins generated by complement or by acute-phase proteins. Fortunately, B lymphocytes exist with specificities for any antigen; although it may take several days or even weeks for a primary antibody response to develop, they ensure that

Table 1.5 Antimicrobial substances produced by phagocytes

Enzymes	Phospholipase A	Breaks down lipid membranes of microorganisms
	Proteinases	Digest protein components of microorganisms
	Lysozyme	Digests peptidoglycan in cell walls, especially Gram-positive bacteria
	DNAase, RNAase	Breaks down nucleic acid (DNA, RNA)
Microbicidal peptides	Defensins	Form ion channels in membranes of microorganisms causing lysis
Reactive oxygen intermediates (ROIs)	Superoxide anion ($O_2^{\bullet-}$)	Very toxic to ingested microorganisms Generates other oxidizing agents
	Hydrogen peroxide (H_2O_2)	Toxic to microorganisms
	Singlet oxygen ($^1O_2$)	Toxic to microorganisms
	Hydroxyl radical ($OH^{\bullet}$)	Toxic to microorganisms
Reactive nitrogen intermediates (RNIs)	Nitric oxide (NO)	Toxic to ingested microorganisms Also reacts with superoxide anion to produce other toxic RNIs
	Nitrogen dioxide (NO_2)	Toxic to microorganisms
	Nitrous acid (HNO_2)	Toxic to microorganisms

any microbes that breach recognition by the innate opsonins are eventually recognized by the receptors of the adaptive system. Moreover, several bacteria have thick polysaccharide capsules that resist innate recognition unless they are first opsonized by antibody. The opsonic and other properties of antibodies are discussed in more detail in the next section.

Once the microorganism has become bound to the surface of a phagocyte it becomes surrounded by the cell membrane and enclosed within a compartment called the **phagosome**. Following phagocytosis, the phagosome undergoes a series of maturational events caused by the fusion of smaller compartments, including **lysosomes** (to produce a **phagolysosome**). Lysosomes contain a lethal cocktail of enzymes and microbicidal peptides that operate to kill and breakdown the contents of the phagolysosome (Table 1.5). Phagolysosomes also become gradually more acidic as they mature, caused by the delivery of a proton pump and the removal of sodium/potassium ATPase. This acidification helps kill ingested microorganisms and provides the optimum pH for the activity of the enzymes. Phagocytosis by neutrophils and macrophages also stimulates a metabolic process called the **respiratory burst**, in which several toxic metabolic by-products of oxygen and nitrogen are produced to assist in the killing process (Table 1.5).

Phagocytes also release the contents of lysosomes by exocytosis to enable extracellular digestion of microorganisms to occur. Digested material is also released by this process. This debris is picked up by actively endocytic professional antigen-presenting cells (APCs) in the skin called **Langerhans cells**, which are essential for the subsequent activation of T cells and development of an adaptive immune response. In response to inflammatory cytokines, Langerhans cells leave the inflamed site via the draining lymph, and migrate through the lymphatic system to the nearest lymph node. During this migration the Langerhans cells lose their endocytic properties and instead gain costimulatory molecules to become potent activators of naive T lymphocytes in the lymph node. In the lymph node they are called **interdigitating dendritic cells**.

T cells that are activated in lymph nodes by interdigitating dendritic cells proliferate and, after a few days, leave via the blood. These cells adhere to activated vascular endothelium, in much the same way as neutrophils did earlier during the acute phase, and infiltrate the site of inflammation. Macrophages are also professional APCs, meaning in essence that they bear class II major histocompatibility complex (MHC) molecules, and can present antigen to CD4+ T cells that enter the site. A subclass of activated CD4+ cells called T_H1 cells (see section 1.6) release cytokines that elevate macrophages to a state of heightened microbicidal and antigen-presenting activity. This process is called **macrophage activation**, and is discussed in section 1.5.2. The respiratory burst is also dramatically increased after macrophage activation by T_H1 cells and enables them to become much more potent killers of ingested microorganisms, particularly those that are adapted to living within the phagosomes of resting macrophages (see Table 1.3).

1.4.3 *The roles of antibody in clearance of extracellular pathogens*

Antibodies are the secreted forms of B-cell antigen receptors and form the humoral arm of the adaptive immune system. These molecules mediate a variety of effector mechanisms that remove invading organisms (Table 1.6). Primary exposure to antigen is relatively slow to elicit specific antibodies

Table 1.6 Functions of antibodies (human) (see reviews by Burton and Woof, 1992; Lamm, 1997)

Isotype	Main functions
IgM	Pentamer, potent activator of complement cascade; the first Ig produced during a primary response; also constitutively expressed as membrane-bound monomer with IgD on B cells as part of BCR* complex
IgD	Constitutively expressed as membrane-bound receptor with IgM on B cells as part of BCR complex
IgG1	Main function is opsonization; also neutralization, ADCC and activation of complement; the major isotype produced during secondary response and found in blood and in tissues; can be transported across placenta
IgG2	Neutralization; found in blood and in tissues; can be transported across placenta
IgG3	Opsonization, neutralization, ADCC and activation of complement; found in blood and in tissues; can be transported across placenta
IgG4	Neutralization; found in blood and in tissues; can be transported across placenta
IgA	Neutralization; transported across epithelia as dimer into secretions
IgE	Degranulation of mast cells; involved in immunity to helminth worms and several allergic diseases

* BCR, B-cell receptor.

because of the need for clonal expansion of the appropriate T_H and B lymphocytes. It may take several days before antibodies appear in the blood, and several weeks before the response undergoes affinity maturation to produce high affinity antibodies. However, a secondary response upon re-exposure to the same antigen elicits the effector mechanisms more rapidly owing to the elevated concentration of serum antibody and the pool of memory B and T_H cells that remain after a primary response.

Neutralization

One of the simplest functions of antibodies is to prevent the attachment of microorganisms and bacterial toxins to receptors on epithelial cells. This process is called **neutralization** (see reviews of virus neutralization by Bachmann

Table 1.7 Fc receptors (human)

Receptor	Cellular expression	Major ligand
FcγRI (CD64)	Monocytes, macrophages, induced on neutrophils by interferon-γ	IgG1, IgG3
FcγRII (CD32)	B lymphocytes, neutrophils, monocytes	IgG1, IgG3
FcγRIII (CD16)	Macrophages, NK cells, neutrophils, eosinophils, Langerhans cells	IgG1, IgG3
FcεRI	Mast cells, eosinophils, basophils	IgE
FcεRII (CD23)	Macrophages, eosinophils, B lymphocytes	IgE
FcαR	Monocytes/macrophages, granulocytes	Polymeric IgA1, IgA2

and Zinkernagel, 1997; Stewart and Nemerow, 1997). Neutralization is performed mainly by IgG, which is the major isotype found in the blood, and IgA found in secretions (tears, saliva, mucus and milk).

Another simple but useful property of antibodies arises from their possession of two identical antigen-binding sites. This enables antibodies to cross-link two antigens simultaneously. This effect is amplified by IgM, which exists as a pentamer (10 binding sites) in its soluble form. In this way, extracellular microbes can become agglutinated into **immune complexes**, which are more readily ingested by phagocytes and entrapped by follicular dendritic cells in secondary lymphoid tissues. Agglutination is particularly efficient if there are repeated copies of the antigen, such as the structural components in the capsid of a virus.

Opsonization

The ability of antibodies to neutralize or agglutinate pathogens does not, in itself, effect their removal. This is performed by accessory cells bearing **Fc receptors** (Table 1.7). These cells include phagocytes (macrophages and neutrophils) which ingest and kill antibody-opsonized microbes, and several granulated cells (mast cells, eosinophils, basophils and NK cells) which are triggered to release preformed components stored in their granules onto the surface of antibody-coated microbes (detailed below). Each Fc receptor is part of a signal transducing complex that communicates the extracellular binding event to the interior of the cell and triggers the effector response. To prevent non-specific tissue damage it is important that triggering only occurs in response to antibody bound to antigen and not free antibody. This is achieved in part by a subtle conformational change in the

Fc region caused by antigen binding, and by the need for Fc receptors to be aggregated on the cell surface for signal transduction to occur. One of the most important functions of antibody in host defence is to coat microbial surfaces to promote uptake by phagocytes bearing Fc receptors (**opsonization**). Studies *in vitro* have shown that macrophages are several hundred-fold more efficient at ingesting bacteria that have been opsonized with IgG than without.

Activation of complement by the classical pathway

During inflammation, increased vascular permeability allows fluid to leave the blood and permeate the site. This fluid contains important components in host defence such as complement, and later, antibodies. In the early stages of inflammation, complement is activated directly by microbial cell walls (the alternative pathway), although as the response progresses and antibodies gradually permeate the site, the cascade becomes activated also by the classical pathway. An outline of this pathway can be found in Figure 1.2.

Degranulation of eosinophils and mast cells

There are size constraints on phagocytosis. Helminth worms, for example, are too large to be ingested by individual cells. Phagocytes may adhere to opsonized surfaces and contribute to their destruction by releasing the contents of their lysosomes onto the surface of the parasite. However, the main effector mechanism appears to be mediated by IgE. Receptors for the Fc region of IgE are found on mast cells, basophils and eosinophils. Mast cells are fragile cells that degranulate in response to tissue injury and are important early initiators of inflammation. Components released by mast cells also trigger muscular contraction (leading to responses such as sneezing and vomiting) and this is thought to be an important mechanism in the expulsion of IgE-coated worms from the gut. Many allergic diseases such as asthma feature the overactivation of this particular system and may represent an unfortunate side effect of having an effective response against worm infestations.

1.5   Responses to intracellular pathogens

Many pathogens replicate in the cytoplasm of infected host cells (Table 1.3). These can be divided into those that reside in the cytosol (which consists of the cytoplasm of a cell excluding the membrane-bound organelles) and those that have adapted to growth within endosomes. Both types of organisms are inaccessible to antibodies and must be destroyed by other means.

1.5.1 Cytosolic pathogens

Pathogens that reside in the cytosol of a cell, such as viruses, can only be destroyed if the cell on which they depend is killed. The major innate defence is lysis by natural killer (NK) cells, and that of the adaptive system is mediated by CD8+ cytotoxic T lymphocytes (T_C cells). More on these cells can be found in reviews by Doherty (1996), Kagi et al. (1996) and Moretta (1997). In the case of viral infection, these effector mechanisms are augmented by the antiviral activities of **interferons** (discussed in more detail in Chapter 3 section 3.2.3).

Natural killer (NK) cells

NK cells are related to T lymphocytes as they differentiate from common progenitor cells. However, these cells lack antigen receptors and the accessory molecules (CD3, CD4, CD8, etc.) that are the hallmarks of T cells. Like CD8+ T_C cells the major function of NK cells is to kill cells infected with viruses and cytosolic bacteria such as *Listeria*. The means by which T_C cells and NK cells kill infected cells is the same, although the means by which infected cells are recognized is different. Both types of cell contain vesicles (or 'lytic granules') that are packed with preformed lytic components called perforins and granzymes. Upon contact with an infected target cell the granules relocalize to the interface and are discharged into the surface of the target cell. Perforins assemble into cylindrical structures within the plasma membrane of the target which allows the granzymes to enter through the polyperforin pore. It is noteworthy that perforin is homologous to the C9 component of the complement membrane attack complex, suggesting their genes evolved from a common ancestor. The granzymes comprise a cocktail of eight or more proteases and esterases. Once inside the target cell these cleave inactive substrates of intracellular signalling cascades leading to the activation of genes for apoptosis. As we will see later, T_C cells can in addition trigger apoptosis through the Fas–Fas ligand pathway, and through the action of tumour necrosis factor-α (TNF-α).

NK cells can identify target cells using their own innate receptors, or via antibodies produced by the B lymphocytes

(**antibody-dependent cell-mediated cytotoxicity** – see below).
The innate receptors have a broad spectrum of activity for
ligands commonly found on transformed cells. Several have
been identified including a C-type lectin that binds to carbohydrate structures on the target cell (reviewed by Ryan
and Seaman, 1997). Killing mediated by this route is regulated by another class of receptor, which in humans is called
the killer inhibitory receptor, or KIR (Colonna, 1997). This
binds to class I MHC molecules and, although also a member of the immunoglobulin gene superfamily, the KIR is distinct from the antigen receptors of T cells. It has been known
for some time that NK cells selectively kill infected cells
that lack surface class I MHC molecules. This is because
the presence of class I on a target cell delivers an inhibitory
signal through the KIR that blocks the NK cell from killing
the target. Many viruses have evolved means for down-regu-
lating the surface expression of class I MHC molecules as a
means to evade recognition by T_C cells. The role of NK cells
is thought therefore to be killing of such cells to limit the
replication of viruses during the early stages of infection
while the T_C cells response is mobilized.

The activity of NK cells is significantly enhanced when
they are exposed to type I interferons released by virus-
infected cells. A similar effect is mediated by IL-12 which is
released by dendritic cells and activated macrophages.

CD8+ cytotoxic T lymphocytes (T_C cells)

Although NK cells are no doubt important in the early stages
of infection, they cannot eliminate viral infection altogether.
This is performed by the cell-mediated arm of the adaptive
immune response. T_C cells recognize virus-infected cells by
the presence of peptides derived from the enzymatic processing of viral proteins that are displayed by class I MHC
molecules on the surface of the infected cell. The receptor
for peptide/MHC is the T-cell antigen receptors (TCR). An
overview of the class I MHC pathway of antigen processing
is given in Figure 1.3. As we will see in Chapter 3 (section
3.2), viruses have evolved numerous strategies to interfere
with this pathway to escape recognition by T_C cells. T_C cells
are also important effector cells in killing macrophages
infected with the intracellular bacterium, *Listeria*. These
bacteria escape the hostile environment of the phagosome
by using a lipase (listeriolysin) to erupt from the phagosome
to the relative safety of the cytosol. However, they then
become accessible to the class I MHC pathway of antigen
processing.

Figure 1.3

Schematic representation of the class I and class II pathways of antigen processing.

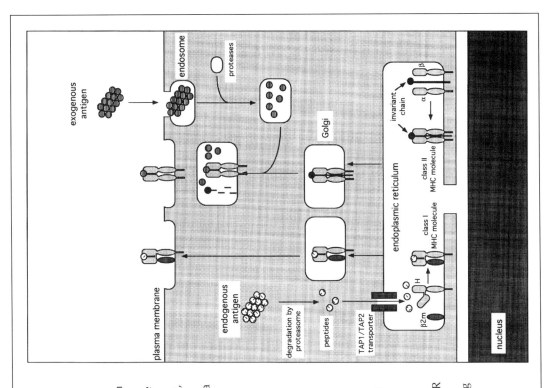

The antigenic universe can be divided into endogenous and exogenous antigens. Those produced in the cytosol include cellular proteins and those produced by cytosolic pathogens such as viruses and *Listeria*. These antigens are degraded in the cytosol into short peptides around 9 amino acids in length by a multisubunit catalytic complex called the proteasome. These are actively transported into the endoplasmic reticulum through an ATP-dependent peptide transporter formed by a TAP1/TAP2 heterodimer. Some of these peptides bind to the peptide-binding cleft of nascent heavy chains of class I MHC molecules, which promotes their assembly with the light chain, β_2-microglobulin (β_2m). Assembly of the trimolecular complex results in its stabilization and export, via the Golgi apparatus, to the cell surface for presentation to the TCRs of CD8+ T_C cells.

Exogenous antigens comprise those that enter the cell from outside by endocytosis (phagocytosis, pinocytosis). These include extracellular and endosomal microorganisms (see Table 1.3) as well as cellular proteins and receptors found in the plasma membrane. These are killed and degraded by enzymes delivered by the fusion of lysosomes. Meanwhile, nascent class II MHC molecules assemble in the endoplasmic reticulum with a chaperone called the invariant chain. Part of the invariant chain occupies the peptide-binding cleft of class II molecules, thereby blocking binding of peptides transported in through TAP1/TAP2. The invariant chain also redirects the export of class II molecules from the Golgi to a compartment of the endocytic pathway called MIIC (MHC class II compartment). Here the invariant chain is digested away by lysosomal enzymes, allowing a peptide derived from processed exogenous antigen to bind in its place. The peptide/class II MHC complex is then transported to the cell surface where it is displayed to the TCR of CD4+ T lymphocytes. Note: only dendritic cells, macrophages and B lymphocytes express class II MHC molecules and can act as antigen-presenting cells for CD4+ T cells.

See reviews by Sant and Miller, 1994; Hahn *et al.*, 1996; Harding, 1996; York and Rock, 1996; Wubbolts *et al.*, 1997. Figure from H. Davies, *Introductory Immunobiology*, Chapman & Hall, 1997, with permission.

T_C cells share the same cytotoxic mechanism involving the release of perforins and granzymes that we have encountered with NK cells. While this mechanism accounts for the bulk of the cytotoxic activity of T_C cells, these cells possess two other means for inducing apoptosis in infected target cells. One is via the Fas–Fas ligand pathway. Fas is found on many cells and its ligation by Fas ligand triggers a signalling cascade that sets apoptosis in motion (Takayama *et al.*, 1995). Fas ligand is expressed on CD8+ T_C cells and T_H1 cells, conferring both with the capacity to kill target cells via this route. T_C cells can also kill targets through the release of cytokines. Activated CD8+ T cells and T_H1 cells release interferon-γ (IFN-γ), TNF-α and TNF-β (lymphotoxin) which together have multiple effects in antiviral immunity. TNF-α and TNF-β have direct cytotoxic effects on cells that bear TNF receptors. These cytokines also activate macrophages making them more potent microbicidal cells (see section 1.5.2).

Antibody-dependent cell-mediated cytotoxicity (ADCC)

Cells infected with viruses sometimes display viral proteins at their surfaces thereby rendering them susceptible to ADCC. This is mediated by NK cells which bear receptors for the Fc regions of IgG1 and IgG3 (CD16 or FcγRIII – see Table 1.7). NK cells are activated when surface CD16 is cross-linked by binding to antibodies on the surface of infected cells. This triggers the release of perforins and granzymes as described earlier. Like the classical pathway of the complement cascade, ADCC is another example of an effector mechanism that can be triggered by either innate or adaptive modes of recognition.

1.5.2 *Endosomal pathogens*

Macrophages are phagocytes that are particularly effective at ingesting and destroying extracellular microorganisms. However, several pathogens have evolved means for living within the vacuoles of resting macrophages (Table 1.3). These include, for example, the bacteria that cause Legionnaires' disease (*Legionella pneumophila*), tuberculosis (*Mycobacterium tuberculosis*), typhoid fever (*Salmonella typhimurium*) and listeriosis (*Listeria monocytogenes*). *Legionella, Mycobacterium* and *Salmonella* alter the nature of the membrane of the phagosome, making it more resistant to fusion with lysosomes. *Mycobacterium* is also able to raise the pH of the phagosome. These organisms can only be killed by enhancing the microbicidal contents of the phagosomes by macrophage activation.

Macrophage activation

As we learned earlier, macrophages release inflammatory cytokines during phagocytosis which activate vascular endothelium as well as causing fever and the release of acute-phase proteins (section 1.4.2). Macrophages are also professional antigen-presenting cells (express surface class II MHC molecules) and are able to present peptides derived from endosomal pathogens to activated CD4+ T lymphocytes (see Figure 1.3) causing the latter to release cytokines. As we will learn in the next section, activated CD4+ cells belong to T_H1 or T_H2 phenotypes, according to the cytokines they produce. The main function of T_H1 cells is to coordinate the effector mechanisms of macrophages, which they do by secreting cytokines that cause macrophage activation. Inflammation triggered in the tissues by antigen-specific T_H1 cells (as opposed to inflammation triggered non-specifically by tissue damage or microbes) is called **delayed type hypersensitivity** (DTH) and is an important form of defence against intracellular pathogens. The main cytokine delivered by T_H1 cells is IFN-γ, although a second signal is first required to induce the expression of IFN-γ receptors on the macrophage. This signal can be provided by the CD40 ligand on the surface of the T_H1 cell, which stimulates the macrophage first through CD40. CD8+ T_C cells and NK cells also produce IFN-γ and can also help to activate macrophages.

The activation of macrophages causes a dramatic increase in the respiratory burst and the production of toxic nitrogen and oxygen metabolites (Table 1.5). Activation also increases the rate of fusion between phagosomes and lysosomes. Together these effects help to kill organisms like *Mycobacterium* that reside within the phagosomes of resting macrophages (see reviews by Kaufmann, 1993; James, 1995; Russell, 1995). Macrophages that are host to particularly resilient organisms become progressively less able to be activated and ultimately unable to clear the infection. During such cases of chronic infection the infected macrophages become enclosed within a sheath of lymphocytes and macrophages called **granulomatous tissue**. Other effects of macrophage activation include an increase in the expression of class II MHC and the T-cell costimulatory molecule, B7.1 (CD80), which allows them to activate naive CD4+ T cells. In addition to inflammatory cytokines, activated macrophages also secrete several

Table 1.8   Changes in macrophages after activation by T_H1

Substances secreted	
IL-1	Inflammatory properties
	Provides costimulation for T-cell activation by antigen
IL-6	Inflammatory properties
	Stimulates haemopoiesis in bone marrow
TNF-α	Inflammatory properties
	Direct cytopathic effect on infected cells
IL-12	Directs differentiation of CD4+ T cells during activation by antigen into T_H1 cells
	Activates NK cells
IFN-α	Induces antiviral resistance in cells
Receptors up-regulated	
CD40	Receptor for CD40L on activated T cells which causes expression of IFN-γ receptors on macrophage
TNF-α receptor	TNF-α secreted by activated macrophages synergizes with IFN-γ from T_H1 cell to induce respiratory burst
B7 molecules (CD80, CD86)	Provides costimulation for T-cell activation by antigen
Class II MHC	With costimulation, promotes activation of naive CD4 T cells by antigen
Other effects of activation	
	Respiratory burst leading to dramatic increase in production of toxic reactive oxygen and nitrogen intermediates

cytokines and other soluble components (Table 1.8), including IL-12, which helps push these newly activated T cells down the T_H1 differentiation pathway (see next section).

1.6   The effector functions of CD4+ T cells

In this final section we will examine the effector functions of CD4+ T cells. The activation of CD4+ T cells is a very stringently controlled process and only occurs in the presence of both antigen (peptide/class II MHC) and costimulatory molecules on the surface of professional antigen-presenting cells. The most potent T-cell costimulatory molecules are CD80 and CD86 (previously called B7.1 and B7.2) and are

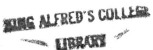

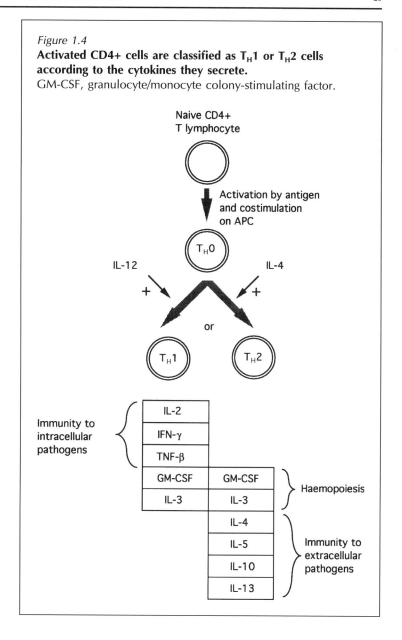

Figure 1.4

Activated CD4+ cells are classified as T$_H$1 or T$_H$2 cells according to the cytokines they secrete.

GM-CSF, granulocyte/monocyte colony-stimulating factor.

expressed mainly on mature (interdigitating) dendritic cells, activated macrophages and activated B lymphocytes. Naive CD4+ T cells can differentiate after activation by antigen into one of several different phenotypes, although the main ones are termed T$_H$1 and T$_H$2 as depicted in Figure 1.4 (see also reviews by Abbas *et al.*, 1996; Mosmann and Sad, 1996). These subsets are defined by the particular cocktail of cytokines they produce, and therefore the effector functions they play in host defence (Table 1.9).

Table 1.9 The functions of T_H1 and T_H2 cytokines (major functions have asterisks)

Cytokine	Effects on target cells	Effect on immune response
IFN-γ (from T_H1, T_C cells)	* Stimulates macrophage activation (respiratory burst)	Enhances killing of intracellular bacteria; promotes inflammation
	* Stimulates elevation of MHC class I and II on many cells	Enhances presentation of antigen to T lymphocytes
	Primes cells to shut down protein synthesis	Enhances resistance of many cells to virus infection
	Stimulates class switching of immunoglobulin to IgG1 and IgG3	Enhances production of opsonins
IL-2 (T_H0, T_H1, some T_C cells)	* Stimulates proliferation of activated T cells	Enhances T-cell mediated immunity (especially T_C cells)
	Stimulates proliferation of B cells	Elevates numbers of APCs
	Stimulates proliferation of NK cells	Enhances immunity to viral infection
TNF-β = lymphotoxin (T_H1, some T_C cells)	* Stimulates macrophage activation (respiratory burst)	Enhances killing of intracellular bacteria
	Killing of tumour cells and infected cells	Enhances immunity to viral infection
IL-4 (T_H2)	* Stimulates proliferation of B cells	Enhances antibody-mediated immunity
	* Stimulates class switching to IgG1 and IgE	Enhances opsonization and immunity to helminth worms
	* Stimulates elevation of MHC class II on B cells	Enhances antigen presentation to T_H2 cells
	Stimulates growth of mast cells	Enhances immunity to helminth worms
IL-5 (T_H2)	Stimulates class switching to IgA	Enhances antibody-mediated immunity
	Stimulates growth of eosinophils	Enhances immunity to helminth worms
IL-6 (T_H2)	Stimulates proliferation of B cells	Enhances antibody-mediated immunity
GM-CSF (T_H1 and T_H2)	Stimulates haemopoiesis of myeloid cells	Increases production of granulocytes (neutrophils, basophils and eosinophils)
	Stimulates differentiation of monocytes	Increases production of macrophages and dendritic cells
IL-3 (T_H1 and T_H2)	Stimulates haemopoiesis	Increases production of granulocytes and mononuclear cells (monocytes and lymphocytes)

1.6.1 T$_H$1 cells coordinate cell-mediated immunity

The signature cytokines of T$_H$1 cells are IFN-γ, IL-2 and TNF-β. The main function of T$_H$1 cells is macrophage activation, which is mediated mainly by IFN-γ secreted by T$_H$1 and cell-surface CD40L. As we saw earlier, macrophage activation promotes their release of inflammatory cytokines and induces a respiratory burst. IFN-γ produced by T$_H$1 also induces immunoglobulin (Ig) class switching in B lymphocytes to IgG1 and IgG3, which are strongly opsonic. Thus, T$_H$1 cells play a major role in coordinating macrophage-mediated immunity.

T$_H$1 cytokines also have other effects that are important in immunity to intracellular pathogens. IFN-γ elevates the expression of several genes in the MHC which leads to enhanced processing of antigens by the class I MHC pathway and presentation to T$_C$ cells. IFN-γ also has a direct antiviral effect by enhancing the resistance of cells to support viral replication (discussed in section 3.2.3). IL-2 produced by T$_H$1 is required for proliferation of T$_C$ cells and by T$_H$1 themselves. TNF-β secreted by T$_H$1 can induce apoptosis and allows T$_H$1 cells to have direct cytopathic activities on infected target cells.

1.6.2 T$_H$2 cells coordinate humoral immunity

The signature T$_H$2 cytokines are IL-4, IL-5 and IL-10. The main role of T$_H$2 cells is to provide cytokines required for immunity to extracellular pathogens. IL-4 is essential for the activation and proliferation of B cells, and later is required for immunoglobulin class switching to IgG1 and IgE. IgG1 is strongly opsonic, while IgE sensitizes mast cells. IL-4 and IL-10 also increase the production of mast cells, whereas IL-5 promotes the growth of eosinophils. Recall that these cells bear Fc receptors for IgE, which trigger degranulation in response to binding IgE-coated helminth worms. T$_H$2 responses are therefore dominant in immunity to helminth worms, and also many allergic diseases through IgE-mediated degranulation of eosinophils and mast cells. IL-4 and IL-10 also increase the expression of class II MHC on B cells, thereby enhancing their interaction with T$_H$2 cells.

Resting B lymphocytes are also antigen-presenting cells, able to internalize antigen captured with their membrane-bound immunoglobulin. Antigen is then broken down in endosomes, as depicted in Figure 1.3, and the peptides exported to the surface by class II MHC molecules, where they are displayed with costimulatory molecules to CD4+ T lymphocytes. Recognition of these peptides by T$_H$2 cells

stimulates them transiently to express CD40L (a potent costimulatory molecule for B lymphocytes) and to release the
cytokines necessary for proliferation and differentiation of
the B cell into a clone of plasma cells (see review by Clark
and Ledbetter, 1994). Notice that this interaction only occurs
between B cells and T cells that have antigen receptors for
the same antigenic structure. This is called **cognate recognition** and it ensures that T-cell 'help' (costimulation and
cytokines) is only delivered to those B cells that need to be
activated.

1.6.3 T_H0 cells differentiate into T_H1 or T_H2

It is now accepted that T_H1 and T_H2 are not separate lineages
of T_H cells but either can arise from a common naive CD4+
precursor. The pathway of differentiation is determined by
signals received by the T cell during the early stages of its
differentiation. Newly activated T_H cells form a heterogene-
ous population of partially differentiated effector cells that
are not yet committed to either pathway. These cells secrete
cytokines characteristic of both T_H1 and T_H2 and are termed
T_H0. However, T_H0 represent an important source of cytokines
required by differentiating B cells. Thus while T_H2 are vital
for protection to metazoan parasites, T_H0 and T_H2 are both
important for immunity to other extracellular pathogens.

A major influence on determining down which pathway
a T_H0 cell will become committed is the presence of IL-12
which promotes differentiation into a T_H1 cell, or IL-4 which
promotes differentiation into a T_H2 cell. Macrophages, dendritic cells and NK cells produce IL-12 during infections
with intracellular pathogens, which tends to push the development of recently activated T_H0 down the T_H1 pathway. In
contrast, IL-4 must be present to induce T_H2 differentiation
instead. T_H0 cells produce small amounts of IL-4 themselves
immediately after activation, although repeated T-cell stimulation is necessary to provide sufficient IL-4 for promot-
ing differentiation along the T_H2 pathway. Other sources of
IL-4 also exist, such as the newly defined subset of CD4+ T
lymphocytes that bear an NK cell marker (NK1.1) which
produce large amounts of IL-4 after activation. NK1.1 CD4+
cells are activated by microbial antigens, although instead
of class II MHC molecules, these cells appear to recognize
antigen in the context of the non-polymorphic class I-like
molecule, CD1 (Bendelac *et al.*, 1997).

As the response progresses, irreversible commitment to
one or other pathway occurs and switching is rare. Indeed,
when one examines the phenotypes of activated T_H cells

Table 1.10 Self-sustaining and cross-regulatory effects of T_H1 and T_H2 cytokines

T_H1 cytokines	
IL-2	Autocrine action on T_H1 cells
IFN-γ	Inhibits T_H2 proliferation in response to antigen
T_H2 cytokines	
IL-4	Promotes differentiation of T_H0 into T_H2
	Antagonizes action of IL-12
	Inhibits macrophage activation (inflammation)
IL-10	Blocks release of IL-12 from dendritic cells
	Inhibits macrophage activation (inflammation)
IL-13	Inhibits macrophage activation (inflammation)

in vivo during an immune response to a pathogen, either a T_H1- or a T_H2-type response predominates. The reasons for this are twofold (Table 1.10). First, once T cells commit to a particular pathway it becomes self-sustaining. T_H1 cells bear IL-2 receptors; therefore the IL-2 they secrete drives their own proliferation in an autocrine fashion. Similarly, IL-4 produced by T_H2 cells amplifies further T_H2 development. The second reason lies in cross-regulatory mechanisms, such that T_H1 cytokines suppress the development of T_H2 and vice versa. For example, IFN-γ produced by T_H1 cells inhibits the proliferation of T_H2 cells in response to antigen. Conversely, IL-4 and IL-10 produced by T_H2 cells antagonize the effects of IL-12 and block its release from dendritic cells, respectively. IL-4 and IL-13 inhibit macrophage activation, whereas IL-10 blocks this and many other macrophage activities.

Ultimately, the type of response that is elicited is vital to host defence. In the main, intracellular infections elicit a T_H1-type response and cell-mediated immunity, whereas extracellular infections elicit T_H2 cells and antibody-mediated reactions. However, mounting an inappropriate response may lead to persistence of the pathogen and possible pathological consequences. The importance of this has been clearly revealed from studies of *Mycobacterium leprae*, an intracellular bacterium that causes leprosy. Some individuals are predisposed to mounting effective T_H1-mediated immunity, whereas others mount T_H2-mediated responses and are unable to clear the infection (discussed in section 2.2.3). The importance of the dichotomy has also been revealed from the study of the protozoan, *Leishmania* (section 4.4). In these examples, host genetic factors probably play a major role in determining which type of response predominates. However, some pathogens (notably some viruses such as the

Epstein–Barr virus) produce homologues of human cytokines which are used to shift the developing immune response for the benefit of the pathogen (see section 3.2.3).

Summary

- Microorganisms that breach the mechanical and chemical barriers of epithelium are exposed to innate and adaptive defence mechanisms. Innate reactions are triggered first. A key initial reaction is inflammation, which can be triggered by mast cell degranulation caused by tissue trauma, or by activation of the alternative complement pathway by microbial surfaces. Tissue macrophages are attracted by chemotactic factors released by mast cells and by by-products of the complement cascade. These cells ingest microbes and release inflammatory cytokines which activate vascular endothelium and recruit neutrophils from the blood to assist in phagocytosis. Opsonins generated by complement coat the microbes and enhance clearance by phagocytes bearing complement receptors. Complement can also lead to the formation of a membrane attack complex in microbial membranes. NK cells are also mobilized early in the response against host cells that become infected with intracellular pathogens.

- Meanwhile, microbial antigens are carried back to draining lymph nodes by dendritic cells or lymph where naive CD4+ T cells are activated. This is the initiation of the adaptive response. CD4+ T cells differentiate into T_H1 or T_H2 cells according to the type of pathogen. Intracellular pathogens such as viruses, intracellular bacteria and protozoa cause T_H1 (inflammatory or DTH) cells to develop. These supply cytokines required for the differentiation of CD8+ T cells into cytotoxic effector cells to kill virus-infected cells. T_H1 cells also produce cytokines required by macrophages to initiate a respiratory burst to kill intracellular bacteria within vesicles. In contrast, extracellular pathogens cause T_H2 (helper) cells to emerge. These produce cytokines required for B lymphocytes to make antibodies against the pathogen. Antibodies are adapter molecules that mediate several effector mechanisms in extracellular fluids (interstitial fluid, lymph, blood and secretions). These include neutralization and immune complex formation, opsonization via Fc receptors on phagocytes, ADCC via Fc receptors on NK cells, triggering complement by the classical pathway, and degranulation of mast cells/eosinophils. Memory is mediated by a residual pool of previously activated T and B lymphocytes that remain after the response subsides.

Study problems

1. What kind of immune responses are appropriate against viruses in (a) the extracellular phase of their life cycle, and (b) after infection of a host cell?
2. How do macrophages kill ingested bacteria and how is this process helped by T_H1 cells?
3. How does the complement cascade help in the removal of invading microbes?
4. With reference to antigen-processing pathways, describe how a virally infected cell preferentially activates T_C cells rather than the production of antibodies.
5. What are the cytokine profiles of T_H1 and T_H2 cells and how do these determine the outcome of the adaptive immune response?
6. Compare and contrast recognition and killing of infected cells by T_C and NK cells.
7. How do helper T cells 'know' to which B cells they must deliver cytokines?
8. In what ways do antibodies help in the removal of invading microorganisms.

Selected reading

Abbas, A.K., Murphy, K.M. and Sher, A., 1996, Functional diversity of helper T-lymphocytes, *Nature*, **383**, 787–793

Ahmed, R. and Gray, D., 1996, Immunological memory and protective immunity – understanding their relation, *Science*, **272**, 54–60

Bachmann, M.F. and Zinkernagel, R.M., 1997, Neutralizing antiviral B cell responses, *Annu. Rev. Immunol.*, **15**, 235–270

Bendelac, A., Rivera, M.N., Park, S.H. and Roark, J.H., 1997, Mouse CD1-specific NK1 T cells: Development, specificity, and function, *Annu. Rev. Immunol*, **15**, 535–562

Burton, D.R. and Woof, J.M., 1992, Human antibody effector function, *Adv. Immunol.*, **51**, 1–84

Clark, E.A. and Ledbetter, J.A., 1994, How B and T cells talk to each other, *Nature*, **367**, 425–428

Colonna, M., 1997, Specificity and function of immunoglobulin superfamily NK cell inhibitory and stimulatory factors, *Immunol. Rev.*, **155**, 127–133

Deitsch, K.W., Moxon, E.R. and Wellems, T.E., 1997, Shared themes of antigenic variation and virulence in bacterial, protozoal, and fungal infections, *Microbiol. Molec. Biol. Rev.*, **61**, 281–293

Doherty, P.C., 1996, Cytotoxic T-cell effector and memory function in viral immunity, *Curr. Top. Microbiol. Immunol.*, **206**, 1–14

Fearon, D.T. and Locksley, R.M., 1996, The instructive role of innate immunity in the acquired immune response, *Science*, **272**, 50–54

Frank, M.M. and Freis, L.F., 1991, The role of complement in inflammation and phagocytosis, *Immunol. Today*, **12**, 333–336.

Goodnow, C.C., 1996, Balancing immunity and tolerance – deleting and tuning lymphocyte repertoires, *Proc. Natl. Acad. Sci. USA*, **93**, 2264–2271

Hahn, Y.S., Yang, B. and Braciale, T. J., 1996, Regulation of antigen-processing and presentation to class-I MHC restricted CD8+T lymphocytes, *Immunol. Rev.*, **151**, 31–49

Harding, C.V., 1996, Class-II antigen-processing – analysis of compartments and functions, *Crit. Rev. Immunol.*, **16**, 13–29

James, S.L., 1995, Role of nitric oxide in parasitic infections, *Microbiol. Rev.*, **59**, 533–547

Kagi, D., Ledermann, B., Burki, K., Zinkernagel, R.M. and Hengartner, H., 1996, Molecular mechanisms of lymphocyte-mediated cytotoxicity and their role in immunological protection and pathogenesis *in vivo*, *Annu. Rev. Immunol.*, **14**, 207–232

Kaufmann, S.H.E., 1993, Immunity to intracellular bacteria, *Annu. Rev. Immunol.*, **11**, 129–163

Kinoshita, T., 1991, Biology of complement: the overture, *Immunol. Today*, **12**, 291–295

Lamm, M.E., 1997, Interaction of antigens and antibodies at mucosal surfaces, *Annu. Rev. Immunol.*, **51**, 311–340

Liszewski, M.K., Farries, T.C., Lublin, D.M., Rooney, I.A. and Atkinson, J.P., 1996, Control of the complement system, *Adv. Immunol.*, **61**, 201–283

Matsushita, M., 1996, The lectin pathway of the complement system, *Microbiol. Immunol.*, **40**, 887–893

Mondino, A., Khoruts, A. and Jenkins, M.K., 1996, The anatomy of T-cell activation and tolerance, *Proc. Natl. Acad. Sci. USA*, **93**, 2245–2252

Moretta, A., 1997, Molecular mechanisms in cell-mediated cytotoxicity, *Cell*, **90**, 13–18

Mosmann, T.R. and Sad, S., 1996, The expanding universe of T-cell subsets: T_H1, T_H2 and more, *Immunol. Today*, **17**, 138–146

Ofek, I., Goldhar, J., Keisari, Y. and Sharon, N., 1995, Nonopsonic phagocytosis of microorganisms, *Annu. Rev. Microbiol.*, **49**, 239–276

Russell, D.G., 1995, Of microbes and macrophages – entry, survival and persistence, *Curr. Opin. Immunol.*, **7**, 479–484

Ryan, J.C. and Seaman, W.E., 1997, Divergent functions of lectin-like receptors on NK cells, *Immunol. Rev.*, **155**, 79–89

Sant, A.J. and Miller, J., 1994, MHC class-II antigen-processing – biology of invariant chain, *Curr. Opin. Immunol.*, **6**, 57–63

Sprent, J., 1997, T cells and memory lapses, *Trends Microbiol.*, **5**, 259–260

Stewart, P.L. and Nemerow, G.R., 1997, Recent structural solutions for antibody neutralization of viruses, *Trends Microbiol.*, **5**, 229–233

Takayama, H., Kojima, H. and Shinohara, N., 1995, Cytotoxic T-lymphocytes – the newly identified Fas (CD95)-mediated killing mechanism and a novel aspect of their biological functions, *Adv. Immunol.*, **60**, 289–321

Turner, M.W., 1996, Mannose-binding lectin: the pluripotent molecule of the innate immune system, *Immunol. Today*, **17**, 532–540

Wubbolts, R., Fernandez-Borja, M. and Neefjes, J., 1997, MHC class II molecules: transport pathways and antigen processing, *Trends Cell Biol.*, **7**, 115–118

York, I.A. and Rock, K.L., 1996, Antigen processing and presentation by the class-I major histocompatibility complex, *Annu. Rev. Immunol.*, **14**, 369–396

2 Bacteria

2.1 Classification of bacteria

Early scientists held the view that life on earth was dichotomous. That is, all living organisms were either plants or animals. However, with the discovery of microorganisms two different primary kingdoms were proposed: the **eukaryotes** (comprising the protozoa, slime moulds, fungi, algae, plants and animals) and the **prokaryotes** (the bacteria). Several other kinds of unicellular organisms were subsequently described, for example the **thermoacidophiles**, that have a form of metabolism that is distinct from prokaryotes and eukaryotes. These organisms were placed into a new primary kingdom called **archaebacteria** (ancient bacteria) and are probably living descendants of the earliest forms of life on Earth. More recently, genetic homologies have been used to study the phylogenetic relatedness of organisms. This is achieved by comparing the sequences of homologous genes, such as the gene for ribosomal ribonucleic acid (rRNA), which is highly conserved across great evolutionary distances. Currently, the tree of life based on rRNA sequence comparisons comprises three domains: the **Bacteria**, the **Eukarya** (corresponding to the old prokaryotes and eukaryotes, respectively) and the **Archaea** (thermoacidophiles and others). Reviews on phylogeny can be found in Woese *et al.* (1990) and Pace (1997).

In a clinical situation, bacteria and viruses are by far the most common causative agents of human diseases. The bacteria are single-celled organisms with both DNA and RNA (which contrasts them with viruses). Unlike eukarya, the chromosomes of bacteria are not enclosed within a nuclear membrane and they have no membrane-bound organelles such as mitochondria, Golgi apparatus or endoplasmic reticulum. A cell wall is usually present which may possess appendages such as pili, fimbriae and flagella. At the simplest level bacteria can be divided into groups depending on their staining characteristics and their morphology, although biochemical, molecular and genetic techniques are also applied.

Morphology

There are three principal morphologies of bacteria that can aid in identification. First are **cocci** (spheres). These can be arranged in chains of cells (such as the streptococci) or in pairs (*Pneumococcus*) or in irregular grape-like bunches (such as staphylococci). These arrangements depend on the cleavage plane during binary fission of a cell into two daughter cells. Division in a single plane gives rise to long chains or pairs, whereas division in two or more planes results in bunches of cells. Second are **bacilli** (rods). These include *Escherichia coli*, *Salmonella* spp., *Pseudomonas* and *Legionella*. These bacteria divide at right angles to their long axis and so do not arrange themselves in a variety of ways. The third morphology is **spiral** or twisted. These are also rod-shaped bacteria that can be spiral (such as *Campylobacter*) or comma-like rods (such as the vibrios).

Surface structures of bacteria

Surrounding the cell membrane of all bacteria (except mycoplasmas) is a rigid protective shell called the **cell wall**. In addition to osmotic protection, the cell wall plays an important function in host–cell interactions and the pathology associated with bacterial infection. Biosynthesis of the cell wall is a major target for some antibiotics such as penicillin which inhibit cell wall synthesis. Mycoplasmas are therefore resistant to such antibiotics because they do not have a cell wall. The cell wall owes its strength to a layer of **peptidoglycan** (Figure 2.1), a gel-like polymer consisting of a backbone of alternating *N*-acetylglucoseamine and *N*-acetylmuramic acid. Peptidoglycan is vulnerable to digestion by **lysozyme**, an enzyme of the innate immune system that cleaves the bond connecting *N*-acetylglucoseamine to *N*-acetylmuramic acid.

The **Gram stain** is perhaps the most important bacteriological stain and is used for the diagnostic identification of microorganisms. Typical Gram-positive cells, such as staphylococci, retain the crystal violet dye after decolourization using ethanol or acetone, which is enhanced by the addition of iodine through the formation of a dye–iodine complex to give a characteristic purple colour. In contrast, Gram-negative bacteria such as *Neisseria* spp. appear to lose the dye–iodine complex after washing and counterstain with different stains such as safranin (giving red or pink). Those which are poorly stained by the Gram stain are referred to as acid-fast stained organisms and include bacteria such as *Mycobacterium tuberculosis*. A more harsh Ziehl–Neelsen staining technique is employed for these and other bacteria that do not bind simple stains and which do not easily

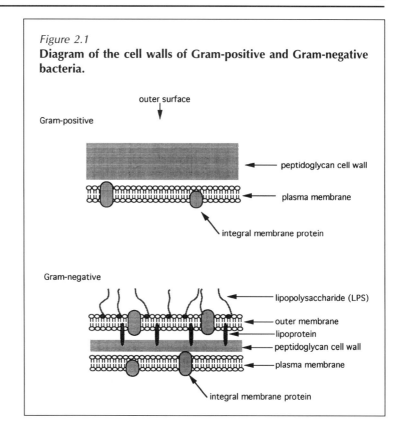

Figure 2.1
Diagram of the cell walls of Gram-positive and Gram-negative bacteria.

outer surface

Gram-positive

← peptidoglycan cell wall

← plasma membrane

← integral membrane protein

Gram-negative

← lipopolysaccharide (LPS)

← outer membrane
← lipoprotein
← peptidoglycan cell wall
← plasma membrane

← integral membrane protein

decolourize by the acid–alcohol wash because of a waxy layer in the cell wall.

The differential staining properties of bacteria correspond with structural components of the cell wall. The cell walls of most Gram-positive bacteria are composed primarily of a thick peptidoglycan layer, which is combined with polysaccharides and a considerable amount of the water-soluble polymer, teichoic acid, covalently linked to the *N*-acetylmuramic acid. The teichoic acids constitute major surface antigens, which lie on the outside surface of the peptidoglycan layer and which are accessible to antibody. The thick layer of peptidoglycan provides good protection against the formation of the complement C5–C9 membrane attack complex, although Gram-positive bacteria are relatively susceptible to digestion with lysozyme.

The cell walls of Gram-negative bacteria do not contain teichoic acids, although the structure is much more complex. The layer of peptidoglycan overlying the plasma membrane is thinner and surrounded by an additional outer lipid membrane that is anchored to the peptidoglycan by lipoproteins. The most important components of this outer membrane are chains of **lipopolysaccharide** (LPS) embedded in it. LPS is a complex molecule consisting of both lipid and carbohydrate which serves to stabilize the outer membrane. LPS is also an **endotoxin** that accounts for the disease symptoms associated with some Gram-negative bacterial infections, such as *Salmonella typhimurium* which causes gastroenteritis. Some species of Gram-negative bacteria also show variability in side chains of the LPS layer called **O antigens**, which allow them to escape recognition by antibodies through antigenic variation (see section 1.2).

The cell wall may also be surrounded by additional structures. Several Gram-positive and Gram-negative bacteria have a thick layer called the **capsule**. Capsules are organized polymers of repeated saccharide residues that are not easily removed and which help mask the underlying antigenic bacterial surfaces. Although the chemical composition varies between different strains and species, most capsules play a major role in the virulence of encapsulated bacteria. Studies of *Streptococcus pneumoniae* in mice, for example, showed that the capsule provides protection against phagocytosis. Normally, mice are killed by infection, but experimental removal of the capsule caused them to lose their virulence. The principal pathogens which cause pneumonia and meningitis in humans also have polysaccharide capsules. These include *Streptococcus pneumoniae*, *Klebsiella pneumoniae*, *Haemophilus influenzae*, *Neisseria meningitidis* and group B streptococci. Sugars are not normally recognized by T lymphocytes so the capsule represents a very weak immunogen. It also resists binding by activated C3a of complement, and provides good protection against the membrane attack complex.

Some anaerobic bacteria (such as *Bacteriodes fragilis*) also produce a polysaccharide capsule called the **glycocalyx** which has been established as a major virulence factor (Brook, 1994). First, these bacteria induce abscesses in the tissues of experimental animals, which have been shown to be inducible by inoculation with purified capsular material alone. This is an anaerobic environment created by infection which is also a hostile niche for the host defence mechanisms. Neutrophils, for example, are not effective phagocytes in abscesses. Secondly, encapsulated anaerobes adhere better to tissue cell surfaces than non-capsulated counterparts. Thirdly, several strict anaerobes are more resistant to phagocytosis than facultative anaerobic organisms, a property that is also mediated by the glycocalyx. Finally, *B. fragilis* appears to be able to interfere with triggering of the alternative pathway of the complement cascade. The major defence against abscess formation by this organism is mediated by T cells. Nevertheless, antibodies are probably useful in defence, because the use of capsular material as a vaccine prevents early bacteraemia in animal models. Although non-encapsulated forms may inhibit the neutrophils migration, these strains seldom cause abscesses.

Several Gram-negative bacteria bear fine, short, hair-like appendages on their surface which are referred to as **pili** (also known as **fimbriae**). These structures are not involved in motility but instead appear to contribute to evasion from host defence. Pili have been implicated in antigenic variation by *Neisseria gonorrhoeae* which is caused by the activation of normally silent pilin genes. In contrast, group A streptococci, which are Gram-positive bacteria, bear protein hairs called **M-proteins** in their outer layer. These are known to be important as strains lacking the M-protein are avirulent. M-proteins have also been shown to prevent complement fixation and thereby confer resistance to phagocytosis mediated by complement-derived opsonins, although the exact mechanism of this mode of evasion is unclear.

Flagella are thread-like structures composed of a single protein, flagellin. Unlike pili, their main function is in motility. Energy needed to rotate the flagellum does not appear to be ATP dependent but instead involves a proton-motive force. Deflagellation of bacteria does not affect the well-being of the cell, and they are quickly regenerated. Motile bacteria can respond to external chemical stimuli by moving either towards the chemical or away from it through positive or negative chemotaxis, respectively. Tactic responses involve not only mechanisms by which bacteria move, but imply the existence of sensing and transducing devices which direct bacteria towards conditions most suitable for survival and multiplication. However, non-motile bacteria such as *Staphylococcus aureus* are also very successful pathogens. *Vibrio cholerae* is monotrichous, meaning it has a single polar flagellum. It is thought to play a role in the initial attachment of the cell to the small intestine and penetration of the intestinal mucus, as non-motile varieties do not succeed in attaching to the epithelium. *Helicobacter pylori* move by means of a bundle of four to seven flagella, which is among a plethora of factors that have been suggested as possible virulence factors of this organism. Each flagellum is enveloped by a relatively acid-resistant membranous sheath that is thought to protect the flagellar filament from disintegration in the gastric lumen.

A number of Gram-positive bacterial pathogens are capable of forming **spores** within their vegetative cells (endospores).

In the environment, spores are resistant to extraordinarily adverse physical and chemical conditions and can remain dormant and viable for many years. When conditions improve, new bacterial cells can emerge from the spores and resume vegetative life. The location of the spore in the vegetative cell varies among species; they may be central (such as *Bacillus anthracis*), subterminal (some clostridia spp.) or terminal (such as *Clostridium tetani*). The terminal spores of certain organisms are sometimes large with swollen sporangium appearing like a drumstick.

2.1.1 *Pathogenesis of bacteria*

Virulence is defined as the relative ability of different strains of a particular species of pathogenic microorganism to cause pathology to its host. The damage occurs because the organism has the ability to either produce toxic proteins (the organism is **toxigenic**) or because it penetrates host tissue, multiplies and spreads (the organism is **invasive**). Virulence can thus be quantified in terms of either the number of organisms or amount of toxin necessary to kill a certain host when administered through an appropriate route. Many pathogenic bacteria produce toxins and other products that damage the host and produce disease. We have already encountered **endotoxins** such as LPS in the cell walls of Gram-negative bacteria. We will now examine the **exotoxins**, which are soluble toxins produced by several bacterial pathogens into the medium in which they are growing.

Exotoxins

The term 'exotoxin' is meant to differentiate these excreted proteins from endotoxins which form an integral part of the cell wall of Gram-negative organisms (Montecucco *et al.*, 1994). However, it is now known that some toxic proteins of bacteria are not normally excreted but are localized in the cytoplasm or periplasm of the bacteria and are liberated during lysis. Exotoxins are produced by many Gram-positive and Gram-negative organisms. They vary considerably in their activities, and the type of host cells or organ they attack. Accordingly, exotoxins may be divided into three categories based on the target site affected:

- **Cytotoxins**, which cause cell death of a variety of cell types by inhibiting protein synthesis. These include *Corynebacterium diphtheriae* which causes diphtheria,

Clostridium difficile which causes pseudomembraneous colitis, and *Shigella* spp. which cause dysentery.

- **Neurotoxins**, which interfere with nerve synapse function. These include *Clostridium tetani* which causes tetanus, and *C. botulinum* which causes botulism.
- **Enterotoxins**, which cause loss of fluid and ion transport across the intestinal mucosa. These include *Vibrio cholerae* which causes cholera, and *Escherichia coli* which causes gastroenteritis.

According to their structure and function, exotoxins can be divided into several types. First, the AB type which is secreted by most exotoxin-producing bacterial species (such as *Shigella dysenteriae*, *C. tetani* and *V. cholerae*). These exotoxins are formed of two subunits, A and B. Subunit A is responsible for the enzymatic activity and, hence, toxicity. On the other hand, the B fragment interacts with specific host-cell receptors. Individually, the A subunit is enzymatically active but lacks binding ability and cell entry capability, whereas the B subunit may bind to the target cell but is non-toxic and biologically inactive. Secondly, there are exotoxins which are able to disrupt cell membranes. These include the α-toxin of *Clostridium perfringens* (which causes gas gangrene) which exhibits a phospholipase activity and is responsible for the killing of phagocytes and causing tissue damage. The third category of exotoxin includes that produced by *Staphylococcus aureus* which causes **toxic shock**. This exotoxin is a **superantigen** which mediates the binding of MHC class II molecules on antigen-presenting cells (APC) to the antigen receptors of CD4+ T lymphocytes. Normally, a CD4+ T cell responds only to a specific complex of class II HLA molecule and antigenic peptide as determined by the antigenic specificity of its T-cell receptor (TCR). However, superantigens cause an indiscriminate association between TCRs and class II molecules that is independent of antigenic peptide. This causes excessive T-cell activation and production of IL-2 which results in a variety of clinical symptoms.

Endotoxins

In contrast to exotoxins, which are soluble proteins usually secreted by growing organisms, endotoxins are complex cell-associated molecules which form part of the outer membrane of Gram-negative bacteria. An important endotoxin is LPS. Although shed by some organisms, endotoxins are mainly released after cell lysis. This can be caused by normal effector mechanisms of the immune system, such as the

membrane attack complex of complement, or during killing
and exocytosis of digested material by phagocytes. Also,
treatment with antibiotics may contribute to the release of
bacterial antigens.

Endotoxins have several direct effects on the host that
cause serious clinical manifestations. First, endotoxins can
trigger inflammation and **fever**. Anything that triggers fever
is called a **pyrogen**. Intradermal injection of small amounts
of endotoxin causes an inflammatory response characterized by infiltration of mononuclear cells (monocytes and
lymphocytes) and, at higher doses, neutrophils. In this
way endotoxins induce fever indirectly by stimulating the
release of inflammatory cytokines from phagocytic cells
(see section 1.4.2). Endotoxins can also cause fever directly,
which can be seen in animal experiments where endotoxins
are administered intravenously. Fever is a prominent feature
in several diseases caused by Gram-negative bacteria, including typhoid fever (*Salmonella typhi*), brucellosis (*Brucella
abortus*), plague (*Yersinia pestis*) and tularaemia (*Francisella
tularensis*). A serious inflammatory condition called **septic
shock** is caused by several Gram-negative organisms when
they are present in large numbers in the bloodstream (bacteraemia or septicaemia). Organisms commonly associated
with septic shock include *E. coli*, *Klebsiella*, *Proteus* and
Pseudomonas aeruginosa.

As alluded to above, inflammatory responses can also be
triggered by bacteria damaged by antibiotics. For example,
patients with active syphilis (caused by the spirochaete,
Treponema pallidum) treated with penicillin develop an
inflammatory response called the **Jarisch–Herxheimer reaction** characterized by syphilitic lesions that may become
more inflamed. This is caused by the release of treponemal
antigens from antibiotic-damaged spirochaetes. These antigens consist of lipid A, which is the toxic portion of the
molecule, and O antigen, which normally extends outwards
from the bacterial surface.

A second important effect of endotoxins is to cause
blood coagulation (clotting) by directly activating factor XII
(Hageman factor) of the clotting cascade. The spreading of
blood clots (**disseminated intravascular coagulation**) is a
frequent clinical complication caused by endotoxins. The
end product of the cascade is the conversion of soluble
fibrinogen into an insoluble gel of fibrin, which obstructs
blood vessels and restricts blood flow to essential organs
including lungs, kidneys, brain and liver. Failure of these
organs and mental symptoms may ensue. In addition, disseminated coagulation depletes the blood of fibrinogen and

platelets. Any trauma may result in uncontrolled haemor-rhaging and organ damage. An example of such a disease includes haemorrhagic manifestations in meningococcal sep-ticaemia, which can have a rapid fatal outcome.

Experimental infusion of animals with endotoxins causes physiological changes which may mimic those seen dur-ing natural infection. Continuous intravenous infusion of a particular dose of endotoxin leads to a state of tolerance to its pyrogenic (fever inducing) effects. This is not seen if it is injected into tissue. Intravenous administration initially causes a reduction in circulating granulocytes (**leucopenia**) which is then followed within a few hours by elevated pro-duction of granulocytes (**leucocytosis**). Metabolic changes also occur, including transient hyperglycaemia followed by hypoglycaemia. This is caused by the increased uptake of glucose by peripheral tissues, and the inability of the liver to control circulating levels. High doses of endotoxin in-duce lethal shock due to hypotension and a fall in cardiac output following the release of vasoactive substances such as histamine. Bacterial endotoxins also activate the comple-ment cascade and stimulate the release of host cytokines. When secreted in high concentrations, both complement and cytokines become toxic. The former cascade activates pha-gocytic processes and cytokines act as signalling molecules that mediate the development of the immune response.

Other pathogenic mechanisms

Many pathogenic organisms produce several substances which do not have a direct toxic effect but which may play an important role in the disease process. *Clostridium perfringens* produces **hyaluronidase** which is an enzyme that breaks down hyaluronic acid, a major component of mucus. This facilitates invasion by the bacilli through host tissues. The breakdown of hyaluronic acids also causes the liberation of carbohydrates which are fermentable (i.e. used as a nutrient source) by the pathogens themselves. Once in the tissues, other products promote the spread of infection, including lecithinase, deoxyribonuclease and collagenase.

Other organisms produce enzymes which are capable of cleaving secretory IgA within the hinge region of the immunoglobulin heavy chain. Not unsurprisingly, these **IgA proteases** are found in organisms that colonize mucosal surfaces where this immunoglobulin is predominantly found, and presumably enhance the ability of such organ-isms to survive on mucosal surfaces. These organisms include *Haemophilus influenzae*, *Neisseria meningitidis*,

N. gonorrhoeae, Streptococcus pneumoniae, S. sanguis and
other mucosal organisms. This strategy alone is insufficient
to protect these organisms from host defences, and nearly
all of the organisms that produce IgA proteases also require
a capsule for virulence (an exception is the gonococcus).

Heat-shock proteins (HSPs) are a third category of bacterial products that contribute to disease. The normal function of HSPs is to act as intracellular molecular chaperones
in the biogenesis of proteins, although they are released by
bacteria when subjected to chemical or physical stresses
(such as low pH or elevated temperature; see Craig *et al.*,
1993). Antibodies to bacterial HSPs are often detected in
individuals with active infection. Humans also have HSPs
that are produced in response to stress, such as bacterial or
viral infections. The amino acid sequences of these human
and bacterial proteins are highly conserved and contain
homologous epitopes which may cause antibodies and T
cells activated against bacterial HSPs to cross-react with self
antigen, perhaps displayed on the surface of infected host
cells, leading to **autoimmune disease**.

Another example is the **listeriolysin O** of the intracellular
bacterium *Listeria monocytogenes*. Normally, this enzyme
allows the bacterium to escape from phagocytic vacuoles
within macrophages into the relative safety of the cytosol
(see section 2.2). Listeriolysin also seems to exhibit a phospholipase C activity and is capable of forming pores in
eukaryotic cell membranes. Other pathogenic streptococci
and staphylococci produce a variety of cytotoxic enzymes
that kill leucocytes, called **leucocidins**. Hydrogen peroxide and ammonia are produced by some *Mycoplasma* and
Ureaplasma spp. as products of their metabolic wastes. These
are toxic and damage epithelia in the respiratory and urogen-
ital systems.

Summary of section 2.1

- Phylogeny is the study of the
  origin of species based on
  evolutionary relationship rather
  than general morphological
  resemblance. Unlike other
  species, it has been difficult
  to trace the evolution of
  microorganisms, mainly because
  of the lack of a reliable fossil

  record. Comparisons of genetic
  material (such as rRNA) of extant
  species have overcome some of
  these problems.

- The cell wall of a bacterium
  mediates initial interactions
  with host cells, protects it
  from immune responses, and

contributes to the virulence of many bacteria. Most bacteria can be classified by differential Gram staining. Gram-positive bacteria have a thick wall of peptidoglycan that provides good protection against complement although it is susceptible to lysozyme. The cell walls of Gram-negative bacteria are more complex; an important component is lipopolysaccharide (LPS). LPS is an endotoxin and also a powerful trigger of inflammation. Many pathogenic bacteria are surrounded by thick polysaccharide capsules which protect them and contribute to the pathogenicity of the organisms. Capsules are also poor immunogens and resist complement.

- Several bacteria secrete exotoxins which block protein synthesis in many cells (cytotoxins), transmission at synapses (neurotoxins) or ion transport by intestinal epithelium (enterotoxins). Endotoxins are toxic components released from bacteria as they multiply or when they are killed. These can cause inflammatory reactions including fever and blood coagulation.

- A variety of other 'virulence factors' are also produced by bacteria that promote their survival or multiplication in the host. These include enzymes (hyaluronidase, IgA protease, listeriolysin O, leucocidins) and heat-shock proteins.

Study problems for section 2.1

1. Describe the bacterial cell-wall structure, and how various structures within and surrounding the cell wall contribute to the virulence of a bacterium.
2. Describe the information that might be obtained by examining a bacterial culture sample under the light microscope.
3. Compare and contrast the mode of action of bacterial toxins.
4. Describe why bacterial heat-shock proteins have been suggested as a cause of autoimmune disease.
5. With reference to named organisms, discuss the role of secretory IgA proteases in disease.

2.2 Intracellular bacteria

The interaction between bacteria and eukaryotic cells is an evolutionarily ancient phenomenon. Indeed, phylogenetic studies teach us that mitochondria are probably descendants of primitive intracellular bacteria that have been adopted by eukaryotic cells because of their ability to produce energy. Such synergism is not always beneficial for bacteria. Several are predated by a variety of eukaryotic cells. Indeed phagocytosis, the means by which macrophages and neutrophils mediate defence against foreign cells and particles, is thought to have evolved from a unicellular feeding mechanism that is still displayed by contemporary mastigophoran (or amoeboid) protozoa. Most multicellular organisms use ingestion by specialized phagocytes to dispose of unwanted cells and debris. In invertebrates phagocytes and other related blood cells also cooperate together to encapsulate invading particles or organisms that are too large to be engulfed by individual cells.

Despite its phylogenetically ancient origins, phagocytosis remains one of the most important defence mechanisms against microbial infection (Finlay and Falkow, 1989; Falkow *et al.*, 1992; Finlay and Cossart, 1997). As such, some species of bacteria, such as *Streptococcus pneumoniae* and *Neisseria meningitidis* have evolved polysaccharide capsules that help resist ingestion by phagocytic cells. Other bacteria have become adapted to an intracellular lifestyle, and promote their own entry into host cells by binding to receptors that trigger phagocytosis. For instance, **invasin**, an outer membrane protein from *Yersinia pseudotuberculosis* triggers phagocytosis and entry of the organism into host cells (Isberg, 1996). Similarly, several other intracellular bacteria (*Legionella*, *Mycobacterium* and *Bordetella*) bind complement receptor 3 (CR3; see section 1.4.1), which is an integrin with a high sequence similarity to invasin receptors. A few Gram-negative bacteria (such as *Bartonella bacilliformis*) exploit erythrocytes as host cells. These cells provide protection from the humoral immune system, they are devoid of intracellular microbicidal defences such as lysosomes, and they have a reasonably long lifespan (100 days).

Once inside the host cell the bacterium has to contend with the hostile environment of the phagosome. Some bacterial species remain within the phagosome, while others escape into the cytosol (*Listeria monocytogenes* and *Shigella* spp.). Those specialized to an intraphagosomal lifestyle evade killing by either inhibiting the phagosome–lysosome fusion (for example, *Mycobacterium tuberculosis* and *Legionella pneumophila*) or by adapting their physiology to the otherwise hostile environment of the phagosome (for example, *Coxiella burnetii* and *Yersinia pestis*). In this section we will examine a few well-characterized intracellular bacteria, namely *Listeria*, *Legionella* and *Mycobacterium*. Additional reviews about intracellular bacteria can be found in Moulder

(1985), Kaufmann (1993), Small *et al.* (1994) and Menard *et al.* (1996).

2.2.1 Listeria monocytogenes

Listeria monocytogenes is a food-borne, Gram-positive, rod-shaped organism that causes infections (**listeriosis**) mainly in individuals with a compromised immune system, although epidemics and sporadic cases of listeriosis also occur in healthy individuals (Farber and Peterkin, 1991). In adult listeriosis, the central nervous system is mainly affected, but it can also cause inflammation of heart valves, and miscarriages during pregnancy. Infections in newborn babies may disseminate in the body causing lesions in the liver or meningitis. Despite modern antibiotic therapy, listeriosis still has a high mortality rate (approximately 36 per cent).

Within two hours after phagocytosis by intestinal macrophages, *Listeria* escapes from the hostile environment of the phagosome by disintegrating the phagosome membrane using a pore-forming toxin called **listeriolysin O**. This enables the bacterium to escape into the relative safety of the cytosol and to replicate. *Listeria* strains that do this are described as **haemolytic** (reflecting their ability to lyse erythrocytes in an *in vitro* assay), whereas strains that are avirulent in humans lack listeriolysin O and are non-haemolytic. Infection is spread between cells by a direct cell-to-cell mode of transmission as depicted in Figure 2.2 (see Tilney and Portnoy, 1989; Kuhn *et al.*, 1990). Dividing intracellular *Listeria* cells become surrounded by cellular actin filaments which develop into a tail-like structure at one pole of the bacterial cell. By a continuous process of polymerization and depolymerization at opposite ends of the tail, the organism is propelled through the cytosol to the plasma membrane. These processes form protrusions at the cell surface that can penetrate into a neighbouring cell and become ingested. Newly infected cells thus contain the bacterium in a two-membrane vacuole which, after lysis by listeriolysin O, releases the organism into the cytosol where it can replicate. Cell-to-cell spread thus allows the organism to disseminate within tissues while remaining hidden from the bactericidal activity of humoral immunity (such as circulating antibodies and complement).

Although antibodies may mediate immunity to *Listeria* in its initial extracellular phase, *Listeria* is a predominantly intracellular organism that requires T-cell mediated responses for effective immunity (see Szalay and Kaufmann, 1996; Bouwer *et al.*, 1997). In the intraphagosomal phase, *Listeria* antigens are exported to the cell surface by class II MHC

Figure 2.2

Diagram of cell-to-cell transmission of *Listeria monocytogenes*.

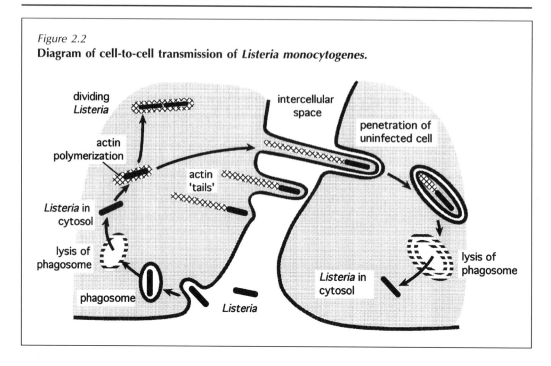

molecules and displayed to CD4+ T$_H$1 cells. In turn these cells activate the microbicidal properties of the infected phagocyte (section 1.5.2). T$_H$1 cells are therefore a major effector lymphocyte in immunity to *Listeria*. After eruption of the bacteria into the cytosol, *Listeria* antigens can then enter the class I MHC pathway instead, and are presented to CD8+ T$_C$ cells. NK cells also mediate the cytotoxicity of cells infected with *Listeria*.

In addition to listeriolysin, there are other factors that contribute to the virulence of *Listeria* (reviewed by Bhunia, 1997). These include **Act A**, a bacterial surface protein which is thought to play an important role in the actin-based motility, and **internalin** (encoded by a chromosomal gene, *inl A*), which is necessary for the entry of *Listeria* into epithelial cells. *Listeria* also produces catalase and superoxide dismutase, which are enzymes that may neutralize the bactericidal activity of ROIs generated by the respiratory burst of infected phagocytic cells.

2.2.2 *Legionnaires' disease bacterium*

An outbreak of a severe, febrile, respiratory illness (legionnaires' disease) occurred during the State American Legion Convention held in Philadelphia in July 1976. The aetiological agent of legionnaires' disease was identified as an airborne bacterium, *Legionella pneumophila*, that gains entry into humans by deep inhalation of infected water droplets. Infections cause pulmonary lesions and severe, often fatal, pneumonia. The disease is associated with a high mortality rate but a low rate of infection. *L. pneumophila* has also been incriminated in an acute, febrile, non-pneumonic illness referred to as Pontiac fever that is characterized by zero mortality and a high infection rate. By and large, *Legionella* is widely spread in our environment and tolerates a wide range of chemical and physical conditions. Although much has been learned about the epidemiology and clinical features of legionnaires' disease and the properties of the causative agent, the immunobiology of the disease and the roles of cellular and humoral immunity are poorly understood.

Intracellular fate and immunity to Legionella pneumophila

Legionella pneumophila is a facultative intracellular pathogen whose natural host is inside human alveolar macrophages (and other phagocytes), although it can also replicate extracellularly on complex media. The bacterium expresses a high-molecular-weight surface protein which is an important antigen that can define different groups of *L. pneumophila* by specific antibodies (serogroups). Antibody to this protein operates as an opsonin which enhances uptake of the organism by mammalian phagocytes. Ironically, it is likely that opsonization by antibodies promotes infection by aiding invasion of host cells. In addition, complement deposited on legionellae may also enhance uptake by opsonization, although some studies show that strains that resist complement deposition are more virulent (Summersgill *et al.*, 1988).

Entry into phagocytes is also dependent on a *Legionella* cell-membrane protein called the macrophage infectivity potentiator (**Mip**; see review of Mip and other virulence factors in Hacker *et al.*, 1993). Mip-negative mutants fail to invade eukaryotic cells and reintroduction of functionally active *mip* gene into *mip*-negative mutant restores virulence. The *mip* gene is also homologous with *mip*-like genes in other intracellular pathogens such as *Neisseria meningitidis, Chlamydia trachomatis* and *Pseudomonas aeruginosa*, in which the Mip protein plays a role in virulence.

Occasionally, internalization of *Legionella* in human monocytes is mediated by a novel type of phagocytosis termed **coiling phagocytosis** (Horwitz, 1984; Rechnitzer and Blom, 1989). Recent studies, however, show that the phenomenon of coiling phagocytosis is independent of bacterial virulence. Once inside the host cell, *Legionella* multiplies in the phagosomes. The pH of the vacuole remains elevated because viable *Legionella* inhibits the fusion of lysosomes with the phagosome and thereby prevents the activation of hydrolytic enzymes. (A similar strategy is used by *Mycobacterium* – see following section.) The membranes of the phagosomes that contain *Legionella* display a novel structure; they become studded with host ribosomes within a few hours after infection and there is some evidence that this causes a significant decrease in total host protein synthesis.

Neutrophils are also important in controlling disease (Fitzgeorge *et al.*, 1988), although precisely how is not clear. This is demonstrated in neutropenic animals (experimentally depleted of neutrophils). Infection of these animals with *Legionella* lowers the dose of organisms necessary to establish infection and leads to increased numbers of bacteria in the lungs and much higher mortality. Moreover, neutropenia did not alter the nature or extent of the pulmonary lesions. Therefore, inflammatory reactions involving neutrophils are not directly responsible for the pulmonary lesions in Legionnaires' disease. The damage is probably caused directly by *L. pneumophila*, in particular by its extracellular enzymes such as proteases.

In addition to the ability to inhibit lysosome–phagosome fusion, legionellae employ other means to thwart host defence. *L. pneumophila* produces an acid phosphatase which blocks superoxide anion generated by the respiratory burst. This organism also produces a metalloprotease which is cytotoxic, tissue-destructive and has phagocyte-inhibitory properties. In addition, *Legionella* produces a heat-stable toxin which impairs O_2 consumption and nicotinamide adenine dinucleotide phosphate (NADPH) turnover during phagocytosis by neutrophils preincubated with the toxin. This presumably benefits the bacterium by reducing the killing ability of neutrophils. *L. pneumophila* also produces a heat-shock protein, iron-superoxide dismutase, and a peptidoglycan-associated protein (which is homologous to lipoproteins of *E. coli* and *H. influenzae*), but their contributions to pathogenicity have not yet been fully established.

Phagocytosis of Legionella *by other eukaryotic cells*

Legionellae are capable of infecting and multiplying within a variety of mammalian and protozoan cell lines (e.g. HL60, HeLa, HEp-2, L929, McCoy, MRC-5, U937 and Vero cell lines and amoebae). The association of *Legionella* with environmental amoebae is well documented. In fact, *L. pneumophila* multiplies inside protozoa and avoids their intracellular

Figure 2.3
Schematic diagram showing events observed when amoebae are infected by *Legionella*-like amoebal pathogens (LLAPs).
Infection is marked by rapid unidirectional or arbitrary motility of intra-amoebal bacteria. During early stages of infection (0–48 h), the nucleus and other cell structures of the amoeba are readily visible. At more advanced stages of infection (beyond 48 h), these structures become less visible or totally indiscernible. Heavily infected amoebae often assume a round rather than the typical irregular shape. The amoebal cell wall eventually ruptures releasing numerous bacteria and the cycle continues. (Figure by N. Adeleke and M.A. Halablab from unpublished data.)

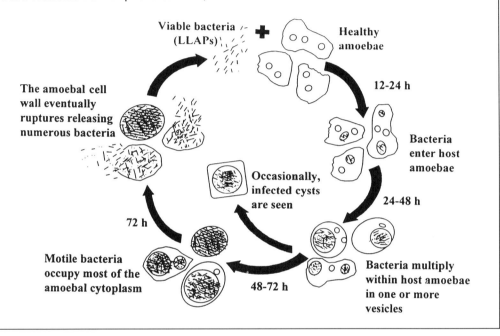

Viable bacteria (LLAPs)

Healthy amoebae

12-24 h

Bacteria enter host amoebae

24-48 h

Bacteria multiply within host amoebae in one or more vesicles

48-72 h

Occasionally, infected cysts are seen

Motile bacteria occupy most of the amoebal cytoplasm

72 h

The amoebal cell wall eventually ruptures releasing numerous bacteria

defences in a similar manner to mammalian phagocytes (reviewed by Halablab *et al.*, 1990). In addition, certain *Legionella*-like amoebal pathogens (**LLAPs**) have not been found to grow, so far, on any microbiological media available, but multiply exclusively inside amoebae. Whereas members of the genus *Legionella*, particularly *L. pneumophila*, are recognized as important aetiological agents of pneumonia, little is known about the clinical relevance of LLAPs. Nevertheless, the majority of the known LLAP strains were originally isolated from sources associated with confirmed cases or outbreaks of legionnaires' disease. In addition, recent phylogenetic analysis shows that almost all the LLAPs known form a coherent cluster with other *Legionella* members in the family Legionellaceae (see Adeleke *et al.*, 1996).

Apart from the mechanism of entry into the host cell, which may differ, the processes involved in the infective cycle of legionellae in amoebae (Figure 2.3) and in mammalian cells are strikingly similar. The ability of *L. pneumophila* to infect epithelial cells is enhanced by prior cultivation of the bacteria in amoebae. Therefore, there may be a connection between the pathogenicity of legionellae for mammalian cells, and their pathogenicity for amoebae (Fields, 1996).

2.2.3 *Mycobacteria*

The majority of the 60 or so species of the genus *Mycobacterium* are harmless, although a few cause serious diseases in humans and other animals. The most serious human diseases are tuberculosis and leprosy, caused by *M. tuberculosis* and *M. leprae*, respectively. Mycobacteria are facultative intracellular pathogens that preferentially infect macrophages and multiply within their phagosomes. Studies with *M. tuberculosis* reveal it survives in the normally hostile environment of the phagosome by reducing fusion between the phagosome and lysosomes. It also prevents the full acidification of the phagosome by reducing the fusion of vesicles containing the proton pump. Precisely how the bacterium controls the fusogenicity of the phagosome in which it resides remains an interesting puzzle and there is considerable interest in identifying the genes that underlie this property (see Clemens, 1996; Collins, 1996).

M. tuberculosis is highly infectious with a high mortality rate of 50 per cent in symptomatic individuals. It is spread from infected hosts by aerosol droplets produced by coughing which are then inhaled by new hosts. The bacteria are particularly resistant to digestion by macrophages, which allows them to persist and leads to the formation of granulomatous tissue and irreversible lung damage. *M. leprae* infections have a lower mortality rate but leprosy is a disfiguring disease that has a particular stigma for humankind.

Several effective drug therapies have been available for human mycobacterial infections for years, and a vaccine (BCG) against tuberculosis was first developed 75 years ago. However, underfunding of eradication programmes and the less than rigorous use of antibiotics have allowed multiple drug resistant (MDR) strains to emerge. Prior to the emergence of MDR strains, the success rate of drug treatment was over 90 per cent. Similarly, the vaccine varies widely in efficacy among different geographical locations and no improvements have been made to the vaccine since it was first developed. This mixture of complacency and poor management has allowed tuberculosis to escalate into a global epidemic that we will probably now never be able to eradicate. Currently, tuberculosis is the second most common infectious disease worldwide, with one-third of the global population infected. Fortunately, only a small minority develop disease, although it has been estimated that tuberculosis will kill 30 million people this decade.

Immunopathology of Mycobacterium

Effective immunity to mycobacteria is mediated by T_H1 cells, predominantly through the activation of antibacterial mechanisms of infected macrophages, and also to a lesser extent via the activation of CD8+ T_C cells (see section 1.5.2 and Flesch and Kaufmann, 1993; Colston, 1996a, b). Although *M. tuberculosis* and *M. leprae* are essentially non-toxic to their host cells, much of the tissue damage associated with these diseases is caused by repeated activation of persistently infected macrophages by T_H1 cells. Macrophages become progressively less responsive to activation and instead become sequestered in sheaths of phagocytes and T lymphocytes called **granulomas**. (In tuberculosis, the granulomas are often called 'tubercles'.) These are small, necrotic, nodular structures within which the bacteria are eventually destroyed. CD8+ T_C cells also probably help to lyse infected macrophages. Non-MHC-restricted T cells have also been implicated in the control of human mycobacterial infections. As granulomas become more numerous, granulomatous tissue develops. The damage is irreversible and leads to gradual loss of normal lung function. Bacteria may also escape the lung in immunodeficient individuals and cause granulomatous tissue in other anatomical sites, including bones and joints, brain, gut, and major organs such as liver and spleen.

Leprosy has become something of a model system for understanding the importance of the T_H1/T_H2 balance in human immune responses to infectious organisms (Modlin, 1994). While effective immunity is mediated by T_H1 cells, antibodies and other responses orchestrated by T_H2-type cells are ineffective against intracellular mycobacteria. Leprosy is a disease that presents in patients as a spectrum of clinical manifestations. At one end of the range is **tuberculoid leprosy** in patients who mount strong T_H1 responses. This is characterized by a high level of protective cell-mediated immunity and the bacteria are effectively removed. However, the acute inflammatory effects of T_H1 cells cause damage to the skin and the loss of peripheral sensory perception caused by nerve damage. This can lead to injuries of the extremities going unnoticed, particularly of the fingers and toes, leading to progressive tissue damage. At the other end of the spectrum is **lepromatous leprosy** in patients who mount strong T_H2 responses and who as a consequence fail to generate effective immunity. Here the bacteria are able to replicate with impunity, particularly in the cooler superficial tissues of the face. Between these two extremes are numerous intermediate forms of the disease, reflecting different balances between bacterial replication and immunological control. Why there should be such a spectrum of immune responsiveness to *Mycobacterium* is not clear, although the inheritance of certain combinations of HLA alleles may be a major influence.

Vaccines and protective immunity

Much can be learned about protective immunity from studying the protective effects of vaccines. The Bacille Calmette–Guérin (BCG) vaccine against *M. tuberculosis* was produced in 1921 and is probably the most widely used vaccine worldwide. The vaccine is an attenuated form of *M. bovis* that was produced by repeated culturing of the bacterium over a period of 13 years in steadily increasing concentrations of bile until it lost its virulence in animals. BCG can elicit both antimycobacterial antibodies as well as CD8+ T_C cells. Because endosomally derived antigens are normally presented by class II MHC molecules to CD4+ T cells, the generation of CD8+ T_C cells by BCG shows that mycobacterial antigens can enter the class I pathway, revealing a novel route of antigen processing (see Figure 1.3).

Globally, some 3 billion people have been vaccinated with BCG since the 1920s, although it has only limited efficacy as a vaccine. A trial in Britain in the 1950s showed that prophylactic immunization of adolescents reduced the incidence of tuberculosis to around 20 per cent of non-vaccinated controls. In other areas of the world, however, the vaccine is far less effective (Fine, 1995). Variations between batches of vaccine, variations in the virulence of different strains of mycobacteria in different geographical locations, the presence of environmental mycobacteria, and genetic variations in the susceptibility to infection among different human populations may all contribute. It has been noticed that previous infection with mycobacteria seems to reduce the

efficacy of the vaccine. Presumably, pre-existing immunity may reduce the ability of the attenuated vaccine strain to
establish an infection of its own, or alternatively the vaccine
may reactivate dormant disease. Moreover, while BCG can
protect newborn babies, it is much less effective at protecting adults, who represent the majority of all cases. Efforts
are underway to modify BCG to improve its efficacy.

Currently, there is no conventional vaccine against leprosy. BCG may offer protection, although the trials in different parts of the world again show that efficacy varies
enormously in different populations. A major hurdle to producing a vaccine against leprosy has been the lack of a
suitable culture system for *M. leprae* organisms. This is
in contrast to *M. tuberculosis*, which can be grown in
macrophage cultures as well as in microbiological media.
The nine-banded armadillo can be used as a surrogate host
for *M. leprae*, although these animals do not keep well in
captivity. It is hoped that the solution will be found by
applying the techniques of recombinant DNA technology.

Engineered vaccines

Efforts are also being made to produce new generations of
vaccines against tuberculosis and leprosy. One approach is
to produce recombinant mycobacterial proteins that can be
used to elicit specific T cells (T_H1 and T_C). Considerable
effort has been spent on identifying the antigens recognized
by *Mycobacterium*-specific CD4+ and CD8+ T cells in patients and experimental animals. However, mycobacteria are
complex microorganisms with many hundreds of different
proteins. Several proteins from *M. tuberculosis* have been
identified and tested for their immunogenicity in animals,
but we are still a long way from having an effective subunit
vaccine. A second approach is to use genetic engineering to
attenuate *M. tuberculosis* or *M. leprae* by deleting the gene(s)
required for their virulence. One candidate is the gene encoding lipoarabinomannan (LAM). LAM is a major component
of the cell wall of most species of *Mycobacterium* that has
several immunomodulatory effects on host cells, particularly macrophages. For example, LAM is a powerful inhibitor of IFN-γ mediated activation of macrophages. The relative
safety of BCG, and its ability to elicit strong cell-mediated
as well as humoral immunity, indicate that BCG would also
make a good vector for the delivery of antigens from other
microorganisms (see Chapter 6).

Summary of section 2.2

- Ingestion by phagocytic cells is a major form of defence against bacteria. Despite their bactericidal property, several bacteria have chosen these cells as the site of replication, while others enter less hostile cells such as erythrocytes. *Chlamydia* and *Rickettsia* are obligate intracellular pathogens, whereas *Legionella pneumophila*, *Mycobacterium* spp. and *Listeria monocytogenes* are facultative intracellular bacteria. These have adopted numerous strategies to avoid the intracellular killing mechanisms. Some species (including *L. pneumophila*, *Mycobacterium*) remain inside the phagosome and inhibit the phagosome–lysosome fusion. In contrast, *L. monocytogenes* escapes the hostile vacuole and multiplies in the cytosol.

- The airborne *Legionella pneumophila* is the causative agent of severe and often fatal pneumonia in humans, legionnaires' disease and non-pneumonic, self-limiting syndrome, Pontiac fever. The infection may also affect the central nervous system, kidneys and gastrointestinal tract. In humans and experimentally infected animals, the organism enters and multiplies within alveolar macrophages. Similarly, legionellae multiply inside amoebae in nature and in laboratory-grown cells.

- The food-borne *Listeria monocytogenes* mainly affects people with suppressed T-cell-mediated immunity. The disease caused by *Listeria* is usually associated with a high mortality rate in adults and neonates in whom the central nervous system, heart and liver can be involved. Miscarriage in pregnant women can also occur. The organism invades host intestinal cells and macrophages by inducing its own endocytosis using a cell-surface protein, internalin. Haemolytic strains escape from the phagosome into the cell cytoplasm and continue to avoid exposure to the humoral immune response by spreading directly from cell to cell.

- *Mycobacterium tuberculosis* and *M. leprae* cause tuberculosis and leprosy, respectively. These organisms survive within the normally hostile phagosomes of macrophages by inhibiting the fusion of lysosomes. Effective immunity is mediated by T_H1 cells that activate antimicrobial mechanisms in infected macrophages (particularly the respiratory burst). In tuberculosis, chronic activation becomes steadily less effective and infected cells instead become encapsulated in granulomas (tubercles) which leads to lung damage. In leprosy, strong T_H1 inflammatory responses lead to clearance of bacteria but also tissue damage (tuberculoid leprosy). In contrast, T_H2 responses are ineffective at clearing infection, although no tissue damage occurs (lepromatous leprosy).

Study problems for section 2.2

1. Compare and contrast the fate of *Listeria monocytogenes* and *Legionella pneumophila* inside eukaryotic cells and the major forms of immune defence against these pathogens.
2. Give an account of the ecology of legionnaires' disease bacterium and *Legionella*-like amoebal pathogens in amoebae and phagocytic cells.
3. Discuss reasons why immune responses to *Mycobacterium tuberculosis* and *M. leprae* can lead to disease.
4. Discuss the 'virulence factors' of *Listeria monocytogenes*.

2.3   Chronic and persistent bacterial infections

As discussed earlier, an infection is defined as the replication of a microorganism within the cells or tissues of a host. **Acute infection** is manifested by the quick appearance of dangerous clinical symptoms whereas **chronic infection** is long lasting, and both are often associated with pathology to the host. In addition, chronic infections may be **latent** when the infective agent assumes a dormant state whilst retaining the capacity to resume pathogenic activity. Other chronic infections may be characterized by a **carrier state** in which an infected individual shows no clinical symptoms, although they continue to release the organisms to infect other susceptible hosts.

There are several bacteria that are able to cause chronic infections in humans. Each display the following characteristics. The immune system is usually unable to eliminate the pathogen completely over a short period of time, either because the pathogen multiplies slowly, or because it is able to hide within anatomical sites secluded from an effective immune response. Moreover, organisms that cause chronic infections generally do not inflict maximal damage to the host, thereby prolonging the survival of both the host and parasite.

2.3.1   *Chlamydial infections*

Chlamydiae are obligate intracellular Gram-negative prokaryotic cells (Beaty *et al.*, 1994). The organisms are responsible for a wide variety of important diseases in animals and humans including trachoma, conjunctivitis, genital and neonatal infections caused by *Chlamydia trachomatis* and psittacosis and pneumonia caused by *C. psittaci* and *C.*

pneumoniae, respectively. Intracellular infection is achieved from a metabolically inactive, infective form of the pathogen, called an **elementary body** (EB). This mediates attachment and invasion of host cells. Inside the cell, EBs undergo morphological changes and differentiate into large reticulate bodies (RBs) which are metabolically active and divide by binary fission to form **inclusion bodies**. After a period of growth and division, RBs redifferentiate into further infective EBs which are released by exocytosis or when the host cell lyses.

Immunopathology of chlamydial infections

Chlamydial infections are frequently asymptomatic and may persist for long periods of time if untreated. Neutralizing antibodies to the organism's outer envelope protein are produced but they are of limited efficacy during the intracellular stages of infection. Very little is known about T-cell responses to these organisms. However, studies with infected cells *in vitro* indicate that IFN-γ may play an important role in controlling *Chlamydia* infection. As we learned in the first chapter, IFN-γ is produced by T_H1 cells when they are stimulated by specific peptide/class II MHC complexes on the surface of infected macrophages. IFN-γ reciprocates by activating antimicrobial mechanisms in macrophages. Low doses of IFN-γ restrict the replication of intracellular *Chlamydia*, although they rapidly re-emerge as viable infectious organisms as soon as the IFN-γ is removed from the cultures. Many species of intracellular bacteria are killed by the toxic ROI generated by the respiratory burst stimulated by IFN-γ. However, *Chlamydia* are resistant to ROIs and are therefore not entirely eliminated from infected cells by the actions of IFN-γ. Instead, the inhibitory effect of IFN-γ on *Chlamydia* replication is due to the activation of a gene whose product is an enzyme that degrades tryptophan. Paradoxically therefore, by being chlamidiastatic, IFN-γ prolongs their survival inside infected cells *in vitro*. This may be a major means by which chronic chlamydial infections are maintained *in vivo*.

During IFN-γ treatment, intracellular forms of chlamydiae with an atypical morphology are produced. A similar effect is seen with penicillin, although why two dissimilar substances should have a similar effect is not clear. Treatment of infected cells with these two mediators also induces the production of chlamydial heat-shock protein (hsp60), which can be detected in immune animals by injecting purified protein into the skin to elicit a characteristic delayed-hypersensitivity response.

C. pneumoniae (first identified in 1986) is responsible for acute respiratory infection in humans and may cause persistent infections. *In vitro* studies indicate that *C. pneumoniae* cells are able to infect and replicate in human smooth muscle cells, macrophages and coronary artery endothelial cells, and a link between chronic infection by *C. pneumoniae* and coronary heart disease has been documented. Moreover in human pathological samples, chlamydial DNA, antigens or EBs can be detected in arterial tissues. The organism contains HSP-like subunits which may lead to autoimmune reactions as discussed above, leading to coronary heart disease (atherogenesis, see Danesh *et al.*, 1997).

2.3.2 Helicobacter *infections*

Until recently, the human stomach has been considered an inhospitable environment for bacterial growth because of its acidic pH. However, in the early 1980s a spiral microaerophilic bacterium (meaning it grows in low oxygen concentrations) was isolated from human gastric mucosa from patients with gastric inflammation. This is a fastidious Gram-negative organism, *Helicobacter pylori*, which has since been established as the major aetiological agent of active chronic gastritis, duodenal and gastric ulcers and more recently has been linked to the development of gastric cancers and heart disease. Other species of *Helicobacter* have subsequently been isolated from the gastric mucosa of several animals. *H. pylori* infections are more prevalent in developing countries where its incidence may be 80 per cent; the incidence is lower in developed countries, around 40 per cent. This makes *H. pylori* one of the most common bacterial chronic infections known.

Although it has not been well established, transmission of infection is thought to be acquired via ingestion through the oral route from oral contact with an infected individual. Once acquired, however, *Helicobacter* infection becomes chronic and may persist for life if untreated with antibiotics. The preferred habitat of the pathogen is the gastric antrum. The spiral morphology, cork-screw motility and microaerophilism of *H. pylori* help the organism to swim rapidly through viscous mucin layers. In contrast, aflagellated strains poorly colonize the stomach in a gnotobiotic piglet model (i.e. devoid of colonizing microbes), indicating that motility is an essential virulence factor. *H. pylori* is non-invasive and seldom penetrates beyond the gastric mucosa. Most cells remain within the mucus overlying the gastric epithelium or adhere to epithelial cells.

Immunopathology of Helicobacter infections

All *H. pylori* isolates identified thus far produce large quantities of **urease**, which may contribute to the pathology of infection. A particular feature of the enzyme is its location on the outer membrane and in the periplasm of the bacterium. *Helicobacter* urease is catalytically efficient (low Km value) at low urea concentrations and breaks down endogenous urea to ammonia. This protects the organism from gastric acidity, but is also toxic to gastric epithelial cells. Urease also acts as a strong proinflammatory agent. Ammonia enhances the recruitment and activation of phagocytes (neutrophils and monocytes), which may lead to neutrophil-dependent gastric mucosal cell injury.

During infection, the host mobilizes both humoral and cellular immunity at the site of infection. Strong T-cell responses to the bacterium are not typically present, but elevated levels of T-cell cytokines (including IL-6, IL-8 and TNF-α) are detected in the gastric epithelium of infected individuals. IL-8 is an important chemokine and activating substance for neutrophils which is also released during chronic gastritis by inflamed epithelial cells. Chronic neutrophil activation could then cause increased free radical formation generated by the phagocyte respiratory burst and may result in mucosal damage. Thus the production of IL-8 in *Helicobacter* infection might be a contributing factor to the immunopathology of peptic ulcers and possibly gastric carcinogenesis. The flagella of the bacterium are highly antigenic and secretory antibodies to *H. pylori* flagella and other surface antigens have also been demonstrated. These reach to and bind to the bacterium *in situ*, but the importance of this in host defence and any counterstrategies (if any) used by the organism remain to be elucidated. Moreover, several epidemiological studies show the association of *H. pylori* antibody titres and coronary heart disease or stroke. The role of the bacteria in these diseases is unclear; the presence of the organism in atheromatous arteries has not been observed, so it has been suggested that autoimmune reactions may trigger atherogenesis.

Another important factor in the pathology is a **vacuolating cytotoxin**, which induces acidic vacuoles in the cytoplasm of infected eukaryotic cells and leads to gastric mucosal ulcers in experimental animals. This substance is produced

by about half of the *H. pylori* strains tested so far. Neutralizing antibodies to the cytotoxin are detectable in the sera
of infected humans. The frequency of cytotoxin-producing
strains isolated from humans is consistently greater among
patients with peptic ulcer disease than among patients with
gastritis only. Approximately 60 per cent of *Helicobacter*
isolates also produce a high-molecular-weight antigenic protein (**CagA**) whose presence correlates strongly with expression of vacuolating cytotoxin activity. Moreover, catalase,
superoxide dismutase, protease, lipase and phospholipase
are also produced by some strains of *Helicobacter*, although
their exact role in disease, if any, is not yet fully understood.

2.3.3 *Immune complex diseases*

As described in Chapter 1 (section 1.4.3), complexes of
antibodies and antigens (immune complexes) are removed
effectively by phagocytic cells or entrapped by follicular
dendritic cells in lymph nodes. However, the chronic production of immune complexes, which often accompanies
infection by several persistent pathogens, leads to overload-
ing of the mononuclear phagocyte system and tissue deposition of complexes. This may lead to pathologies called **type
III hypersensitivity reactions**.

The source of immune complexes (ICs)

There are several sources of ICs. First, they can be caused
by low grade infections with persistent bacteria (such as
with α-haemolytic viridans streptococci and staphylococcal
infective endocarditis), by protozoa (such as *Plasmodium
vivax*) and by viruses (such as hepatitis virus). These infections lead to a prolonged antibody response and to chronic
IC formation, which become deposited in the tissues resulting in IC diseases. Secondly, in patients with autoimmune
diseases such as systemic lupus erythematosus (SLE), in
which there is a continued production of autoantibody to a
self antigen, IC disease is a frequent complication. Thirdly, in
farmer's lung disease, caused by actinomycete moulds such
as *Aspergillus fumigatus*, there are circulating antibodies
that are produced following repeated exposure to mouldy
hay. In this case, ICs are formed at the body surface, in the
lungs following repeated inhalation of antigenic material
from the moulds. Finally, most human malignant tissues
express tumour-specific antigens that can be recognized by
the immune system. Tumour cell necrosis or secretion from

cells may result in the shedding of tumour antigens into the circulation which may combine with antibodies and result in circulating ICs (Salinas and Hanna, 1985).

Immune complex hypersensitivity also can develop as a result of the passive transfer of antiserum for preventing certain bacterial infections. As observed at the end of the last century when injections of horse antitoxin serum were administered to provide passive immunity in the treatment of diphtheria and tetanus, a disease called **serum sickness** sometimes ensued. The sickness is not related to the anti-toxin content of the serum since it can also be produced in response to normal horse serum or serum from other animals. Instead the foreign serum proteins, which are themselves antigens, stimulate antibody production. These antibodies then combine with circulating antigens to form small soluble ICs. These circulate for several days and form inflammatory lesions where they are deposited. The symptoms include painful swelling of the joints (arthritis), renal failure, skin lesions (vasculitis) and fever.

ICs trigger inflammation and tissue damage by neutrophils

Tissue-trapped ICs trigger activation of the classical pathway of complement activation which leads to the production of C3a and C5a. Recall from Chapter 1 (Table 1.4) that these possess anaphylatoxic and chemotactic characteristics which increase vascular permeability and attract neutrophils. Phagocytosis of particularly large complexes is difficult and the neutrophils are more likely to release their lysosomal enzymes to the extracellular fluid by exocytosis. Damage of the tissue may then occur, as depicted in Figure 2.4. If these enzymes are released into the circulation or tissue fluids, they are likely to be neutralized by serum enzyme inhibitors. However, if the phagocyte is in close proximity to the fixed complexes, the enzyme inhibitors will be excluded and damage of the underlying tissue is likely to occur. ICs can also activate blood platelets through their Fc receptors, which leads to aggregation and microthrombus formation and hence a further increase in vascular permeability.

Removal, deposition and persistence of ICs

Phagocytic cells of the liver (Kupffer cells), spleen and lungs are strategically situated and normally remove immune complexes. Whereas small ICs can circulate for long periods,

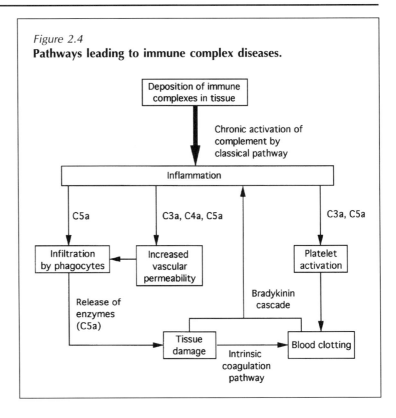

Figure 2.4

Pathways leading to immune complex diseases.

larger complexes are removed by the liver within a few minutes. Therefore, factors which affect the size of the complexes are likely to influence their persistence and rate of removal. For example, defects of the immune system that lead to the production of low affinity antibodies may result in the formation of smaller complexes which persist and may consequently cause IC disease.

The increase in vascular permeability during inflammation is perhaps the most important factor for tissue deposition of ICs. There are several potential contributors to the release of vasoactive amines, including complement and activated mast cells and basophils.

In various diseases ICs seem to home to particular organs. In patients with SLE the kidney is the main target for deposition, whereas in rheumatoid arthritis the joints are the principal target. ICs are inclined to deposit in sites where there is high blood pressure. For example, in the glomerular capillaries in the kidney the blood pressure is approximately four times that of most other capillaries. If the pressure is reduced, IC deposition is also reduced. Other haemodynamic processes such as blood turbulence may also invoke deposition of ICs. It is also possible that the antigen in the complex provides the organ specificity. The strong affinity of DNA for the basement membrane collagen of the glomerulus could lead to the deposition of DNA/anti-DNA antibody complexes in the kidney of patients with SLE where these antibodies are such a noticeable feature. Moreover, bacterial endotoxins that cause cell damage can cause the release of DNA which binds to glomerular basement membranes. Anti-DNA antibody is then produced by activation of B lymphocytes and is bound by the fixed DNA leading to local IC formation. In mouse models of SLE there is a class switch of anti-DNA antibodies from predominantly IgM to IgG2a that occurs as the mice age. The switch occurs earlier in females than in males and coincides with the onset of renal disease, indicating that the class of antibody is important in the tissue deposition of ICs.

2.3.4 *Infections caused by newly emerging and re-emerging pathogens*

Newly emerging bacterial pathogens are defined as bacteria that have not been previously identified, whereas re-emerging bacteria include those that have acquired resistance to antimicrobial therapies and have became important opportunists with increased virulence or pathogenic properties (Krause, 1992; Ihler, 1996; Anderson and Neuman, 1997). Selected examples of these bacteria are summarized in Table 2.1. Counted among the newly emerging pathogens are viable non-culturable bacteria and the infectious proteins or **prions** whose recent emergence has revealed a novel form of infectious disease aetiology.

Table 2.1   Representative list of emerging and re-emerging bacterial pathogens

Bacillus subtilis
Bartonella bacilliformis
Campylobacter
Enterococci
Escherichia coli (enterohaemorrhagic *E. coli*)
Helicobacter pylori
Legionella
Listeria monocytogenes
Mycobacterium tuberculosis
Mycoplasma fermentans
Salmonellae
Spirochaetes
Staphylococci
Streptococci
Vibrios

Summary of section 2.3

- Chlamydial infections affect individuals of different age groups ranging from neonates to adults. Diseases include trachoma, conjunctivitis, genital and neonatal infections, psittacosis and pneumonia. Some of these infections have been associated with serious complications including coronary heart diseases. Responses by T and B cells are largely ineffective, although IFN-γ has chlamydiastatic properties which may exacerbate persistence.

- *Helicobacter pylori* infections in humans are one of the most common bacterial infections known. The organism is adapted to surviving in the hostile acidic niche of the stomach by penetrating the superficial mucosa and by producing urease. Damage to the mucosa by urease can lead to gastritis and ulcers, and *Helicobacter* has also been implicated in gastric cancers and heart disease.

- Immune complex diseases are caused by chronic exposure to antigens, such as after administration of animal sera (serum sickness), bacterial infection (such as acute post-streptococcal glomerulonephritis), autoimmune diseases (such as SLE) and environmental microorganisms (such as farmer's lung). Once formed, immune complexes can deposit in tissues leading to activation of complement and the production of chemotactic agents. These cause the migration of neutrophils to the tissue to attempt to phagocytose the immune complexes. These cells then are stimulated to degranulate and release their enzymes extracellularly, leading to tissue injury.

- During the past two decades, noticeable changes in the occurrence of infectious diseases (bacterial, viral, fungal and protozoan) throughout the world have emerged. The emergence of new microbial agents, and the re-emergence of infections previously believed to be controlled, threatens the well-being of all populations.

Study problems for section 2.3

1. Explain the paradoxical effect of IFN-γ during *Chlamydia* infections.
2. Discuss the life cycle of Chlamydia in eukaryotic cells.
3. Give a detailed account of the gastric ecology of *Helicobacter pylori*. Explain the possible mechanisms that lead to tissue damage.
4. Define immune complex diseases and discuss the roles bacterial infections play in the formation of these complexes.

Selected reading

Books for background reading

Hormaeche, C.E., Penn, C.W. and Smyth, C.J., 1992, *Molecular Biology of Bacterial Infection: Current Status and Future Perspectives*, Soc. Gen. Microbiol., Symposium 49, Cambridge: Cambridge University Press

Mims, C.A., 1987, *The Pathogenesis of Infectious Disease*, 3rd edn, London: Academic Press

Mims, C.A., Playfair, J.H.L., Riott, I.M., Wakelin, D., Williams, R. and Anderson, R.M., 1993, *Medical Microbiology*, London: Mosby

Northfield, T.C., Mendell, M. and Goggin, P.M., 1993, Helicobacter pylori *Infection: Pathophysiology, Epidemiology and Management,* London: Kluwer Academic

Prescott, L.M., Harley, J.P. and Klein, D.A., 1998, *Microbiology*, 4th edn, Boston, Mass: WCB/McGraw-Hill

Salinas, F.A. and Hanna Jr, M.G., 1985, *Immune Complexes and Human Cancer, Contemporary Topics in Immunobiology*, **15**, New York: Plenum

Salyers, A.A. and Whitt, D.D., 1994, *Bacterial Pathogenesis: A Molecular Approach*, Washington: ASM Press

Literature cited

Adeleke, A., Pruckler, J., Benson, R., Rowbotham, T., Halablab, M.A. and Fields, B., 1996, *Legionella*-like amoebal pathogens – phylogenetic status and possible role in respiratory disease, *Emerg. Infect. Dis.*, **2**, 225–230

Anderson, B.E. and Neuman, M.A., 1997, *Bartonella* spp. as emerging pathogens, *Clin. Microbiol. Rev.*, **10**, 203–219

Beaty, W.L., Morrison, R.P. and Byrne, G.I., 1994, Persistent chlamydiae: from cell culture to a paradigm for chlamydial pathogenesis, *Microbiol. Rev.*, **58**, 686–699

Bhunia, A.K., 1997, Antibodies to *Listeria monocytogenes*, *Crit. Rev. Microbiol.*, **23**, 77–107

Bouwer, H.G.A., Barry, R.A. and Hinrichs, D.J., 1997, Acquired immunity to an intracellular pathogen: immunologic recognition of *L. monocytogenes*-infected cells, *Immunol. Rev.*, **158**, 137–146

Brook, I., 1994, The role of incapsulated anaerobic bacteria in synergistic infections, *FEMS Microbiol. Rev.*, **13**, 65–74

Clemens, D.L., 1996, Characterization of the *Mycobacterium tuberculosis* phagosome, *Trends Microbiol.*, **4**, 113–118

Collins, D.M., 1996, In search of tuberculosis virulence genes, *Trends Microbiol.*, **4**, 426–430

Colston, M.J., 1996a, The cellular and molecular basis of immunity against mycobacterial diseases, *J. Appl. Bacteriol.*, **81** (Supplement), 33–39

Colston, M.J., 1996b, The molecular basis of mycobacterial infection, *Molec. Aspects Med.*, **17**, 385–454

Craig, L.A., Gambill, B.D and Nelson, R.J., 1993, Heat-shock proteins: molecular chaperones of protein biogenesis, *Microbiol. Rev.*, **57**, 402–414

Danesh, J., Collins, R. and Peto, R., 1997, Chronic infections and coronary heart disease: is there a link? *Lancet*, **350**, 430–436

Falkow, S., Isberg, R.R. and Portnoy, D.A., 1992, The interaction of bacteria with mammalian cells, *Annu. Rev. Cell Biol.*, **8**, 333–363

Farber, J. and Peterkin, P., 1991, *Listeria monocytogenes*, a food-borne pathogen, *Microbiol. Rev.*, **55**, 476–511

Fields, B.S., 1996, The molecular ecology of legionellae, *Trends Microbiol.*, **4**, 286–290

Fine, P.E.M., 1995, Variation in protection by BCG: implications of and for heterologous immunity, *Lancet*, **346**, 1339–1345

Finlay, B.B. and Cossart, P., 1997, Exploitation of mammalian host cell functions by bacterial pathogens, *Science*, **276**, 718–725

Finlay, B.B. and Falkow, S., 1989, Common themes in microbial pathogenicity, *Microbiol. Rev.*, **53**, 210–230

Fitzgeorge, R.B., Featherstone, A.S.R. and Baskerville, A., 1988, Effects of polymorphonuclear leucocyte depletion on the pathogenesis of experimental Legionnaires' disease, *Br. J. Exp. Pathol.*, **69**, 105–112

Flesch, I.E.A. and Kaufmann, S.H.E., 1993, Role of cytokines in tuberculosis, *Immunobiology*, **189**, 316–339

Hacker, J., Ott, M., Wintermeyer, E., Ludwig, B. and Fischer, G., 1993, Analysis of virulence factors of *Legionella pneumophila*, *Zbl. Bakt.*, **278**, 348–358

Halablab, M.A., Richards, L. and Bazin, M.J., 1990, Phagocytosis of *Legionella pneumophila*, *J. Med. Microbiol*, **33**, 75–83

Horwitz, M.A., 1984, Phagocytosis of Legionnaires' disease bacterium (*Legionella pneumophila*) occurs by a novel mechanism: engulfment within a pseudopod coil, *Cell*, **36**, 27–33

Ihler, G.M., 1996, *Bartonella bacilliformis*: dangerous pathogen slowly emerging from deep background, *FEMS Microbiol. Lett.*, **144**, 1–11

Isberg, R.R., 1996, Uptake of enteropathogenic *Yersinia* by mammalian cells, *Curr. Top. Microbiol. Immunol.*, **209**, 1–24

Kaufmann, S.H.E., 1993, Immunity to intracellular bacteria, *Annu. Rev. Immunol.*, **11**, 129–163

Krause, R.M., 1992, The origin of plagues: old and new, *Science*, **257**, 1073–1078

Kuhn, M., Prevost, M.C., Mounier, J. and Sansonetti, P.J, 1990, A nonvirulent mutant of *Listeria monocytogenes* does not move intracellularly but still induces polymerisation of actin, *Infect. Immun.*, **58**, 3477–3486

Menard, R., Dehio, C. and Sansonetti, P.J., 1996, Bacterial entry into epithelial cells: the paradigm of *Shigella*, *Trends Microbiol.*, **4**, 220–226

Modlin, R.L., 1994, T_H1–T_H2 paradigm-insights from leprosy, *J. Invest. Dermatol.*, **102**, 828–832

Montecucco, C., Papini, E. and Schiavo, G., 1994, Bacterial protein toxins penetrate cells via a four-step mechanism, *FEBS Lett.*, **346**, 92–98

Moulder, J.W., 1985, Comparative biology of intracellular parasitism, *Microbiol. Rev.*, **49**, 298–337

Pace, N.R., 1997, A molecular view of microbial diversity and the biosphere, *Science*, **276**, 734–740

Rechnitzer, C. and Blom, J., 1989, Engulfment of the Philadelphia strain of *Legionella pneumophila* within pseudopod coil in human phagocytes: comparison with other *Legionella* strains and species, *APMIS*, **97**, 105–114

Small, P.L.C., Ramakrishnan, L. and Falkow, S., 1994, Remodeling schemes of intracellular pathogens, *Science*, **263**, 637–639

Summersgill, J.T., Raff, M.J. and Miller, R.D., 1988, Interactions of virulent *Legionella pneumophila* with human polymorphonuclear leukocytes, *Med. Pathol.*, **5**, 41–47

Szalay, G. and Kaufmann, S.H.E., 1996, Functional T cell subsets in mycobacterial and listerial infections: lessons from other intracellular pathogens, *Curr. Top. Microbiol. Immunol.*, **215**, 283–302

Tilney, L.G. and Portnoy, D.A., 1989, Actin filaments and the growth, movement, and spread of the intracellular bacterial parasite, *Listeria monocytogenes*, *J. Cell Biol.*, **109**, 1597–1608

Woese, C.R., Kandler, O. and Wheelis, M.L., 1990, Towards a natural system of organisms: proposal for the domains Archaea, Bacteria, and Eucarya, *Proc. Natl. Acad. Sci. USA*, **87**, 4576–4579

3 Viruses

3.1 Classification of viruses

Viruses have several characteristics that distinguish them from other microorganisms:

- Virus particles have no metabolic or biosynthetic properties, nor contain any membrane-bound organelles such as ribosomes or mitochondria. Viruses are entirely dependent on invading a prokaryotic or eukaryotic host cell in order to replicate. Viruses therefore are often described as obligate intracellular parasites.
- Viruses are smaller than prokaryotic and eukaryotic cells, ranging in size from parvoviruses (22 nm) to the poxviruses (around 230×270 nm). Viruses can only be seen by electron microscopy and not by light microscopy.
- Unlike prokaryotic and eukaryotic cells which contain both RNA and DNA, viruses contain a genome of one kind of nucleic acid, either DNA or RNA. DNA viruses have double-stranded DNA (except parvoviruses which are single stranded), whereas RNA viruses have single-stranded RNA (except reoviruses which are double stranded). Single-stranded RNA viruses are either **positive stranded** and can be translated directly into protein-like mRNA, or **negative stranded** and must first be transcribed by a viral transcriptase into a complementary positive strand before translation.
- The genome of viruses is surrounded by a protein shell (**capsid**) consisting of repeating units (**capsomers**) constructed from a small number of different polypeptides. Most capsids have two basic structural symmetries (Figure 3.1): 20-sided or **icosahedral** symmetry (e.g. polioviruses, herpesviruses) or **helical** symmetry (e.g. influenza viruses). The nucleic acid genome plus the capsid is termed the **nucleocapsid**.
- Some viruses consist of a naked capsid (such as papillomaviruses, poliovirus), while others are surrounded by a lipid membrane called the **envelope** (such as herpesviruses and influenza virus). Viral envelopes are acquired when newly assembled nucleocapsids are released through the nuclear membrane (herpesviruses) or plasma membrane (influenza virus) of infected cells by a process called **budding**. Envelopes usually bear

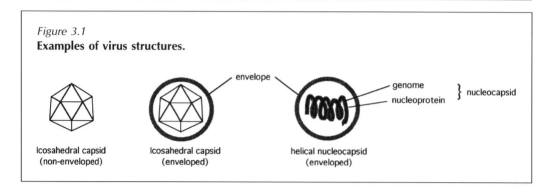

Figure 3.1
Examples of virus structures.

embedded proteins of host cell or viral origin. The nucleocapsid plus envelope (if present) is a complete virus particle called a **virion**.

Viruses are classified according to several criteria (Table 3.1), including the type of nucleic acid in the genome (DNA or RNA); whether the genome is linear, circular or segmented; the polarity of the genome (positive or negative); the morphology of the capsid (icosahedral, helical or complex); and whether an envelope is present. Moreover, strains within a given species can be discriminated according to the specificity of antibodies. If a particular antibody is neutralizing, all strains recognized by it are termed a **serotype**.

The replication cycle of a virus can be divided into a sequence of discrete events:

- **Adsorption**; the attachment of the extracellular virus particle to the surface of the host cell. Adsorption is usually mediated by the binding of a capsid or envelope protein to one or more specific receptor(s) on the surface of the infected cell (Table 3.2).
- **Penetration**; the entry of the capsid through the plasma membrane into the cytosol. This may occur at the cell surface or through the membrane of an endocytic compartment. Enveloped viruses gain entry by fusion of their envelopes with the plasma membrane.
- **Uncoating**; the breakdown of the capsid and release of the viral genome into the cytoplasm.
- **Transcription**; the production of viral mRNA, which often requires enzymes carried in with the nucleocapsid.
- **Translation**; the production of viral polypeptides from viral mRNA using cellular translation machinery.
- **Replication**; the production of new viral genomes. Replication of DNA virus genomes may require host cellular enzymes although some viruses (adenoviruses, poxviruses, herpesviruses) encode their own DNA polymerases.

Table 3.1 Classification of human viruses

Family	Genome	Morphology	Envelope	Virion transcriptase	Examples	Symptoms
Parvoviridae	ss DNA	Icosahedral	No	No	Parvovirus	
Poxviridae	ds DNA	Complex	Yes	No	Variola Vaccinia	Smallpox
Herpesviridae	ds DNA	Icosahedral	Yes	No	Herpes simplex virus (HSV) Varicella-zoster virus (VZV) Human cytomegalovirus (HCMV) Epstein–Barr virus (EBV)	Cold sores, genital herpes Chickenpox, shingles Infectious mononucleosis; lymphoma
Adenoviridae	ds DNA	Icosahedral	No	No	Adenovirus	Gastroenteritis; respiratory infections
Papovaviridae	ds DNA	Icosahedral	No	No	Papillomavirus Polyomavirus	Skin and mucosal warts; cancers
Hepadnaviridae	ds DNA	Icosahedral	No	Yes (DNA to RNA)	Hepatitis B virus	Hepatitis; hepatocellular carcinoma
Reoviridae	ds RNA (segmented)	Icosahedral	No	Yes (RNA to RNA)	Rotavirus	Gastroenteritis
Paramyxoviridae	ss RNA⁻	Helical	Yes	Yes (RNA to RNA)	Human parainfluenza virus Measles virus Mumps Respiratory syncytial virus	Parainfluenza Measles Mumps Respiratory infections
Orthomyxoviridae	ss RNA⁻ (segmented)	Helical	Yes	Yes (RNA to RNA)	Influenza virus	Influenza
Arenaviridae	ss RNA⁻	Helical	Yes	Yes (RNA to RNA)	Lassa virus Lymphocytic choriomeningitis virus	Lassa fever Lymphocytic choriomeningitis

Table 3.1 Cont'd

Family	Genome	Morphology	Envelope	Virion transcriptase	Example	Symptoms
Rhabdoviridae	ss RNA⁻	Helical	Yes	Yes (RNA to RNA)	Rabies virus	Rabies
Bunyaviridae	ss RNA⁻ (segmented)	Icosahedral	Yes	Yes (RNA to RNA)	Bunyavirus	CNS infections Haemorrhagic fevers
Picornaviridae	ss RNA⁺	Icosahedral	No	No	Poliovirus Rhinovirus Hepatitis A virus	Poliomyelitis Common cold Hepatitis
Flaviviridae	ss RNA⁺	Icosahedral	Yes	No	Hepatitis C virus Yellow fever virus	Hepatitis; hepatocellular carcinoma Yellow fever
Togaviridae	ss RNA⁺	Icosahedral	Yes	No	Rubella virus	Rubella (causes birth defects)
Coronaviridae	ss RNA⁺	Icosahedral	Yes	No	Coronavirus	Gastroenteritis and respiratory infections
Retroviridae	ss RNA⁺	Icosahedral	Yes	Yes (RNA to DNA)	Human immunodeficiency virus Human T lymphotropic virus I, II	AIDS Leukaemia
Filoviridae	ss RNA⁺	Helical	Yes	Yes (RNA to RNA)	Ebola virus	Haemorrhaging, fluid loss, shock
Calciviridae	ss RNA⁺	Icosahedral	No	No	Hepatitis E virus	Hepatitis

Table 3.2 Host cell receptors for human viruses

Virus	Viral receptor attachment protein[1]	Host cell receptor	Distribution of host cell receptor	Normal function of host cell receptor[2]
Epstein–Barr virus (EBV)	gp340	CD21 (CR2)	B lymphocytes and follicular dendritic cells	CR2 (complement receptor 2) binds C3d which is opsonic and coats microorganisms; CD21 also a component of BCR complex
Human immunodeficiency virus-1 (HIV-1)	gp120	CD4 plus coreceptor (see below)	Helper T cells (also macrophages, dendritic cells)	CD4 operates with TCR as coreceptor for class II MHC
T-trophic strains		CxC-4	T cells	Receptor for chemokines IL-8, G
M-trophic strains		CCR5	Macrophages and lymphocytes	Receptor for chemokines RANTES, MIP-1α, MIP-1β
Rhinovirus group				
Major (91 serotypes)	VP1/VP2	CD54 (ICAM-1)	Widespread	Intercellular adhesion; ligand for LFA-1
Minor (10 serotypes)	VP1/VP2	Low density lipoprotein receptor	Widespread	
Influenza A virus	Haemagglutinin	Cell surface structures containing sialic acid[3]	Widespread; apparent specificity for structures on respiratory epithelium	Imparts negative charge to cells

Table 3.2 Cont'd

Virus	Viral receptor attachment protein[1]	Host cell receptor	Distribution of host cell receptor	Normal function of host cell receptor[2]
Measles virus	H protein	CD46	Widespread	MCP (membrane cofactor protein): receptor for complement C3b and C4b which allows their degradation by factor I
Polio virus	VP1/2	CD155	Monocytes, macrophages, CNS neurons	Polio virus receptor, normal function unknown
Coxsackie virus	VP2	CD55	Widespread	DAF (decay accelerating factor) binds complement C3b and disassembles C3/C5 convertase

[1] gp, glycoprotein.

[2] BCR, B-cell receptor; TCR, T-cell receptor; RANTES, Regulated upon Activation, Normal T cell Expressed and presumably Selected; LFA-1, leucocyte function-associated antigen-1.

[3] Sialic acid is also known as *N*-acetyl neuraminic acid (NANA).

RNA viruses replicate their genomes with virus-encoded RNA polymerases (e.g. poliovirus, influenza virus). Retroviruses are unique RNA viruses in that their genomes are reverse-transcribed into DNA using viral reverse transcriptase and are then integrated into the host cell genome (**provirus**). Replication of retroviral RNA is therefore via the integrated proviral DNA.

- **Assembly**; the encapsidation of newly replicated viral genomes within the structural (capsid) proteins to produce new virus particles.
- **Egress**; the release of progeny virus from the infected cell, which may also be the stage at which the virus acquires its envelope.

3.1.1 *Pathology of virus infections*

Different viruses have a variety of effects on host cells that can lead to disease symptoms. Many viruses are **lytic**, meaning that after replication within a host cell they burst or lyse the cell as they exit. For example, varicella (chickenpox virus) and herpes simplex are viruses that lyse infected cutaneous epithelial cells. The tissue trauma associated with host cell lysis often leads to a localized inflammatory response which is a key event in initiating an immune response. This is also responsible for many of the disease symptoms associated with viral infections. Other viruses cause infected cells to fuse. Examples include the measles virus and the human immunodeficiency virus. The latter causes multiple fusion events resulting in the formation of large, multinucleate cells called **syncytia**. Other viruses can cause infected cells to become tumour cells (discussed in section 3.5). These include human papillomaviruses which are associated with epithelial tumours, and Epstein–Barr virus which is linked to nasopharyngeal carcinoma and Burkitt's lymphoma.

3.2   Viral immune evasion strategies

Viruses use a remarkable array of strategies to thwart the immune system. Many RNA viruses (e.g., rhinovirus, influenza) utilize antigenic variation as a means of escape, primarily because of their generally higher rates of mutation. A similar strategy is used by the retrovirus, HIV. Other viruses are more antigenically stable and use direct means to subvert immune responses. As a general rule, viruses with large genomes (e.g. the poxviruses, herpesviruses) produce homologues to host cellular proteins that modulate the regulation and effector mechanisms of immune responses. The list of evasive strategies outlined below is not complete but a selective representation of some of the better understood examples. Many other examples along similar lines have been described, and new examples are being reported regularly. Concise overviews of this subject can be found in Gooding (1992) and McMichael (1993, 1997).

3.2.1 *Antigenic variation*

Antigenic variation is an escape strategy used by several different microorganisms. All are able to exist in multiple, antigenically distinct strains to remain one step ahead of a developing adaptive immune response. Rhinovirus (the common cold virus) provides a good example of antigenic variation; this virus exists in over 160 distinct serotypes in human populations, each defined by the specific neutralizing antibodies elicited during infection. Not until a person has been exposed to all of the different serotypes does that person become completely immune to rhinovirus infection. Another example is influenza virus, which has become a paradigm for understanding the molecular details of antigenic variation (discussed in more detail in section 3.3).

Both rhinovirus and influenza virus depend on infecting non-immune (naive) hosts and must move from host to host quickly in order to survive. However, other viruses may change their antigenic structures *during* an infection. This ensures that as an immune response develops there will emerge a small number of variants of the original strain that are not recognized by currently activated lymphocytes. An example of this is HIV, which can at any one time exist in several dozen different strains within a single infected individual (discussed in section 3.4).

These are examples of evasion of antibody-mediated immunity. However, there is mounting evidence for antigenic variation within the targets of CD8+ cytotoxic T lymphocytes (T_C cells) (McMichael, 1993; Koup, 1994). Studies of epitopes from Epstein–Barr virus presented by the HLA-A11 allele have revealed a rare example of the selective pressure exerted on the evolution of microorganisms by T cells (de Campos-Lima *et al.*, 1993). The dominant epitope of the EBNA4 antigen is amino acid residues 416–424 presented by A11. This epitope is well conserved in most strains of EBV carried by Caucasian and African populations. In these populations the frequency of A11 ranges from 0 to 11 per cent of the population. However, in China and Papua New Guinea the A11 allele is present in over 50 per cent of the population. Precisely why the frequency is elevated is not clear, but may be because A11 is an important allele in protecting humans against a particular life-threatening pathogen (or pathogens) indigenous to China and Papua New Guinea. The interesting point is that, in these populations, a strain of EBV predominates that differs from the isolates found in Caucasian and African populations by having an amino acid substitution within the EBNA4 epitope located in critical A11-binding anchor positions. Laboratory studies have shown that these substitutions prevent these particular epitopes from binding to A11 and therefore are not presented to the antigen receptors of T_C cells. This observation strongly suggests that the selection pressure imposed by the immune system can lead to the selection of epitope-loss mutants. Naturally, the polymorphic nature of the MHC allows other alleles to present epitopes of EBV and thereby uphold an effective immune response. None the less, this does show that T_C cells can also exert selective pressure on genetically stable DNA viruses like EBV, as well as upon the more variable RNA viruses such as influenza and rhinovirus.

3.2.2 *Interference with antigen processing*

As we learned in the first chapter, CD8+ T_C cells recognize complexes of short viral peptides and class I MHC molecules displayed on the surface of virus-infected cells (Figure 1.3). The surface expression of class I molecules is often reduced on cells infected with viruses, and in several cases this has been shown to be due to active interference of the class I antigen-processing pathway by the virus (see Table 3.3 and review by Hengel and Koszinowski, 1997). The evolution of such strategies by viruses aids in escape from recognition by T_C cells, and clearly demonstrates the importance of this particular effector mechanism in antiviral immunity.

Adenoviruses

Adenovirus (Ad) is a non-enveloped, double-stranded DNA virus with an icosahedral capsid. Ads are classified according to antigenic properties into 49 serotypes, which are organized into six groups, A–F, according to DNA sequence homology. In humans they usually infect mucosal epithelial cells lining the respiratory and gastrointestinal tract, although infections of the eye and bladder can also occur. A

Table 3.3 Viral proteins that interfere with antigen presentation by class I MHC molecules

Virus	Viral protein	Effect
Adenovirus 2	E3/19K	Arrests transport of class I heavy chains in ER*
Adenovirus 12	?	Down-regulation of genes for TAP, proteasome and class I MHC molecules
Herpes simplex virus 1 and 2	ICP47	Blocks peptide transport into ER by TAP1/TAP2
Epstein–Barr virus	EBNA-1	Internal repeat blocks processing by proteasome
Cytomegalovirus	pp65	Phosphorylates viral IE protein and blocks its processing by proteasome
Cytomegalovirus	gp24	Retrotranslocation of class I MHC heavy chains from ER to cytosol
Cytomegalovirus	gp32/33	Arrests transport of class I heavy chains in ER
Cytomegalovirus	gp33	Retrotranslocation of class I MHC heavy chains from ER to cytosol
Cytomegalovirus	gp69	MHC class I heavy-chain homologue that may inhibit killing by NK cells

* ER, endoplasmic reticulum.

cell-surface receptor by which Ad gains entry to host cells has not been identified. Symptoms of human infection range from mild to severe, and infections are occasionally fatal in immunocompromised patients.

Although infections can persist for months, Ad is usually cleared completely by the immune system. Mice are also susceptible to human Ad infection although the virus is unable to replicate in mouse cells. Although there is no evidence that adenoviruses cause tumours in humans, Ad2 and Ad12 are tumourigenic in rodents. In early infection, four early regions (*E1–E4*) are transcribed. These consist of genes required for transcriptional activation of other genes and for DNA replication. By 7 h after infection, five late genes (*L1–L5*) are transcribed which encode the capsid proteins required for viral assembly. The growth-transforming properties of the virus have been localized to products of the *E1A* and *E1B* transcription units. The *E3* region generates nine different mRNA transcripts that are translated into polypeptides ranging in size from 6.7 to 19 kDa. This region is non-essential for viral replication although it encodes several polypeptides important for evading host immunity (discussed below). Ad has also been engineered in the laboratory for use as a gene delivery vehicle for gene therapy (see section 6.2.3).

Although not the natural host for Ad, mouse cells have proved a useful model for the study of tumourigenicity and evasion of T_C cells. Infection of mouse cells with the tumourigenic Ad (Ad2 and Ad12) causes a dramatic clearing of class I MHC molecules from the cell surface, thereby rendering the infected cell invisible to T_C cells (see reviews by Burgert, 1996; Hayder and Müllbacher, 1996). Interestingly, Ad5 fails to down-regulate class I MHC on mouse cells and is consequently non-tumourigenic in mice.

The mechanisms by which Ad2 and Ad12 down-regulate class I have turned out to be different. In Ad2 this property has been pinpointed to a 19 kDa polypeptide from E3 (called **E3/19K** or gp19). E3/19K is a glycoprotein that is expressed in large amounts during early infection. It is translated with a leader sequence, thereby enabling it to enter the endoplasmic reticulum (ER). This is the first compartment in the pathway for cellular proteins destined for export to the cell surface. Within the ER, the E3/19K protein binds specifically to nascent class I MHC molecules. E3/19K has a di-lysine motif at its C-terminus (**ER-retentional signal**) that blocks transport of itself and bound MHC heavy chain to the cell surface. The structural details of the association between E3/19K and class I MHC molecules have not been fully worked out. However, E3/19K probably interacts with the polymorphic regions of class I (that is, surrounding the peptide-binding cleft) because some mouse class I alleles bind well to E3/19K whereas other alleles do not.

In contrast, Ad subgroups A and F lack E3/19K, yet these viruses are still able to down-regulate class I MHC early after infection. Work with Ad12 (group A) shows that this virus cripples the class I MHC processing pathway by instead interfering with the expression of several important genes simultaneously (Rotem-Yehudar *et al.*, 1996). The expression of TAP1, class I MHC heavy chains and β_2-microglobulin is reduced (mRNA levels 2–40-fold less than normal), whereas expression of TAP2 and the proteosome polypeptides LMP2 and LMP7 are barely detectable after infection (mRNA levels reduced over 100-fold). Precisely how the virus interferes with multiple genes is not yet clear but it may be by targeting a common regulatory element.

Herpesviruses

The family Herpesviridae consists of a family of diverse viruses, classified into three families, α, β and γ, according to their host cells and genetic relatedness (Table 3.4). In

Table 3.4   The Herpesviridae

		Primary infection	Reactivation
α-Herpesviridae	Herpes simplex virus 1 (HSV-1)	Cold sore (fever blisters)	Cold sore
	Herpes simplex virus 2 (HSV-2)	Genital herpes	Genital herpes
	Varicella-zoster virus (VZV)	Chicken pox (varicella)	Shingles (zoster)
β-Herpesviridae	Cytomegalovirus (CMV)	Infectious mononucleosis-like disease	Retinitis Colitis Pneumonitis
	Human herpes virus 6 (HHV6)	Exanthum subitum	?
	Human herpes virus 7 (HHV7)	?	?
	Human herpes virus 8 (HHV8)	Kaposi's sarcoma	?
γ-Herpesviridae	Epstein–Barr virus (EBV)	Infectious mononucleosis (glandular fever)	? Lymphoma

humans, initial or 'primary' infection with herpesviruses normally occurs in the first decade of life. These viruses are famed for causing life-long latent infections that are resistant to elimination by the immune system. Such individuals are called **carriers**. Periodically there are outbreaks of viral reactivation in which replication and shedding of viruses occurs. These may occur when the host immune system is compromised in some way. Usually the site of primary infection by a herpesvirus is different to the site in which latent infection is established. Paradoxically, while herpesviruses are able to resist the immune system they are also dependent on a healthy immune response for their survival, as primary or secondary infections in severely immunocompromised individuals can sometimes be fatal.

To persist within a host for life, and to be able to replicate at sufficient levels to allow transmission to new hosts, the herpesviruses have evolved several different strategies to thwart the immune system. The down-regulation of class I MHC molecules by herpesviruses to escape recognition by T_C cells is one such mechanism (see reviews by Burgert, 1996; Davis-Poynter and Farrell, 1996; Hill, 1996).

Primary infections of HSV occur in the skin, with HSV-1 having a preference for the tissue around the mouth and HSV-2 favouring the genital epithelium. These cause cold sores (fever blisters) and genital sores, respectively. These cutaneous infections are sites in which viral replication occurs. Herpesviruses are lytic viruses, which is the basis of the tissue damage seen in the lesions. Immediately after infection, fibroblasts show a rapid down-regulation of surface class I MHC molecules. The viral protein responsible for this effect has been identified as **ICP47** (Hill *et al.*, 1995). This is a small (9.6 kDa) cytosolic protein that binds with high affinity to the cytosolic face of the TAP1/TAP2 transporter complex. This completely blocks the transport of processed antigenic peptides into the endoplasmic reticulum. In the absence of peptides, newly synthesized class I MHC molecules fail to assemble with β_2-microglobulin and are not exported to the cell surface. The blocking of TAP by ICP47 therefore prevents the display of viral and other peptides to the antigen receptors of T_C cells. Some viruses are transported through neurons into the neural cell bodies located in the dorsal root ganglia where they establish a non-replicative, latent infection where no viral proteins are expressed. Here the virus hides from the immune system by virtue of its quiescent state and because nerve cells are virtually devoid of surface class I MHC molecules.

Another herpesvirus, human cytomegalovirus (HCMV), has evolved a sophisticated array of mechanisms for evading cell-mediated cytotoxicity. The first of these is mediated by the viral matrix protein called **pp65** which enters the infected cell with the virus particle (Gilbert *et al.,* 1996). This protein is a kinase whose function is to phosphorylate a major viral transcription factor that is encoded in the intermediate/early (IE) region of the viral genome. Phosphorylation of the IE protein diverts it from processing and presentation by the class I MHC pathway, although precisely how is unclear. The result is protection of the host cell from killing by T_C cells able to recognize IE-derived antigenic peptides.

Because pp65 enters the cell with the virion, it is preformed and able to exert its protective effect first, before the other mechanisms that require viral gene expression become operational. These subsequent mechanisms are mediated by viral genes, **US2**, **US3**, and **US11**, which together down-regulate the surface expression of class I MHC molecules. US3 encodes gp32/33 which has an ER retentional signal and arrests the transport of newly synthesized class I heavy chains in the ER, in much the same way as Ad E3/19K described above. Meanwhile US2 and US11 gene products (gp24, gp33) cause the heavy chains to be degraded within minutes after they have been synthesized. To do this, HCMV exploits a quality control process the cell routinely uses to destroy abnormal proteins. Normally, cellular polypeptides destined for export to the cell surface are extruded during translation into the lumen of the ER (a process called

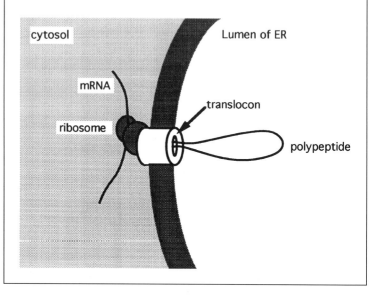

Figure 3.2
The translocation of nascent polypeptides into the endoplasmic reticulum through the translocon.
Retrotranslocation of nascent MHC heavy chains is caused by adenovirus US2 and US11 gene products (see Wiertz *et al.*, 1996).

translocation) through a 'pore' in the ER membrane called the **translocon** (Figure 3.2). The translocon is a cylindrical structure consisting of three to four copies of a complex called Sec61 consisting of three subunits, α, β and γ. Once inside the ER the polypeptides undergo several post-translational modifications, including glycosylation, folding, disulphide bond formation, and assembly with other polypeptides. Any polypeptides that are misfolded or fail to assemble properly are arrested from progressing to the Golgi *en route* for the cell surface, and are instead translocated back out through the translocon into the cytosol. This is thought to be controlled by specific chaperones whose function is to bind to abnormal proteins and escort them back into the cytosol. Once in the cytosol the abnormal polypeptides are rapidly deglycosylated and ubiquitinylated, which targets them for degradation by the proteasome. HCMV exploits this retrotranslocation mechanism as a means for escaping T_C-cell recognition. Both US2 and US11 encode glycoproteins that are translocated into the ER during synthesis. Here they specifically associate with newly synthesized (nascent) class I MHC heavy chains. This triggers the retrotranslocation of class I heavy chains back into the cytosol, possibly by mimicking the actions of cellular chaperones that cause the dislocation of abnormal proteins. The heavy chains are then deglycosylated, ubiquitinylated and degraded (Wiertz *et al.*, 1996).

Encoded in a different part of the HCMV genome is another important gene, **UL18**. This encodes gp69 which is homologous (i.e. shares a similar amino acid sequence) to the human class I MHC heavy chain (Beck and Barrell, 1988). Possibly the virus 'captured' the human gene from its human host at some point during its evolution. Studies *in vitro* showed that gp69 is able to assemble with human β_2-microglobulin (β_2m), which is the light chain of the class I MHC heterodimer. Initially it was thought that its function was to sequester β_2m from human class I MHC heavy chains, thereby blocking assembly of normal class I molecules and transport to the surface. However, HCMV mutants lacking UL18 are still able to down-regulate class I molecules from infected cells. It is now known that the gp69/β_2m heterodimer is able to bind self peptides and becomes transported to the cell surface in much the same way as conventional class I MHC molecules do. This complex is non-functional for recognition by T_C cells. Instead its role is thought to protect infected cells from natural killer (NK) cells. As we learned in Chapter 1, NK cells have evolved to kill cells that lack surface MHC class I molecules, but are inhibited from killing through killer inhibitory receptors (KIRs) that bind class I molecules. The down-regulation of class I by the actions of US2, US3 and US11 as described above would, although protecting them from T_C cells, render them susceptible to NK lysis. The function of UL18 may therefore be to engage KIRs on NK cells and inhibit lysis.

Yet another herpesvirus, Epstein–Barr virus (EBV), utilizes a different mechanism to evade T_C-cell recognition, although in contrast to the above examples, it is designed to protect the virus during latent infection rather than during the lytic (replicative) stages of infection. (See section 3.5.1 for more details on EBV infection.) Replication of EBV occurs in epithelial cells of the oropharynx. These become infected through the transfer of virus shed in the saliva of another infected individual. Primary infections in childhood are usually asymptomatic and the oropharyngeal infections are rapidly cleared by the immune system. However, a proportion of circulating B lymphocytes also become infected as they traffic through infected epithelium. It is in the B lymphocytes that latent, non-replicative infection is established. Although infected B lymphoctes do not support viral replication, they act as a reservoir of infected cells that can re-infect the oropharynx as they periodically traffic

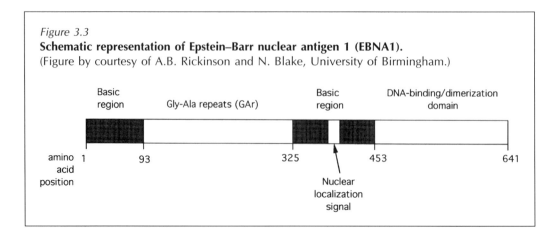

Figure 3.3
Schematic representation of Epstein–Barr nuclear antigen 1 (EBNA1).
(Figure by courtesy of A.B. Rickinson and N. Blake, University of Birmingham.)

through. This leads to recurrent bouts of viral replication and shedding of virions into the saliva.

Several 'latent' genes are expressed in B cells. One of these, EBNA1, has a special motif of glycine–alanine repeats (GAr, depicted in Figure 3.3) that has been found to protect the protein from the class I MHC antigen-processing pathway (Levitskaya *et al.*, 1995). Evidence for this was discovered by engineering the EBNA1 gene in the laboratory. For example, inserting the coding sequence for a known T_C-cell epitope into the EBNA1 gene protects the epitope from being recognized by specific T_C cells. Similarly, insertion of the GAr into a different antigen such as the EBNA3B (which is normally a target antigen for EBV-specific T_C cells) greatly reduces recognition of the EBNA3B antigen. The reasons behind this strategy are not clear. However, the principal function of EBNA1 is the maintainance of the viral genome. Protecting this protein from recognition by T_C cells may therefore be vital to the survival of the virus and lead to its persistence in infected cells.

3.2.3 *Cytokine blockade*

Cytokines play many immunoregulatory roles in the effector phases of immune responses. In particular, the cross-regulatory activites of T_H1- or T_H2-type cytokines ensure that an immune response polarizes into a predominantly cell-mediated or antibody-mediated response as it progresses. Several viruses have 'acquired' homologues of human cytokine or cytokine receptor genes that they use to manipulate or disrupt the normal cytokine network (Spriggs, 1994). Other cytokines such as TNF-α have direct antiviral activity by being able to cause lysis of infected cells, whereas the interferons engender a state of resistance to viral infection in uninfected cells. These too have become the subject of counterstrategies by viruses.

Some viruses interfere with the T_H1/T_H2 balance

Epstein–Barr virus (EBV) and some related viruses have acquired a homologue of the human IL-10 gene called **BCRF-1** (Moore *et al.*, 1990). The predicted amino acid sequence of the EBV homologue is 84 per cent identical with human IL-10 and the viral protein shares many of the same effects as its human counterpart. Human IL-10 is produced by T_H2 cells whose main role is the suppression of T_H1 cells (section 1.6.3). This results in the down-regulation of IFN-γ synthesis by T_H1 cells, while at the same time driving the proliferation of activated B lymphocytes. Viral IL-10 probably serves to help EBV escape the many antiviral activites of IFN-γ (Table 1.9), while providing more B lymphocytes as potential host cells for infection. Recently, the equine herpes virus (EHV), which is related to EBV, has also been shown to have an IL-10 homologue.

Some viruses interfere with inflammation

IL-1, IL-6 and TNF-α produced by activated macrophages cause both local and systemic inflammatory effects (section 1.4.2). The importance of inflammatory processes in the clearance of viral infections is evident from the strategies evolved by different viruses to block the effects of these cytokines. Vaccinia virus (VV) is a poxvirus that has evolved two independent mechanisms to block the activities of IL-1 (Alcami and Smith, 1995). One involves the production of a soluble viral homologue of the IL-1β receptor, called **B15R**. This protein has 25 per cent amino acid identity with the type I human IL-1 receptor, and 33 per cent identity with the type II receptor. B15R is liberated in prodigious amounts by infected cells and it has the property of specifically neutralizing any IL-1β. This has the effect of reducing the inflammatory and pyrogenic (fever-causing) effects of IL-1, and is presumably important for the survival of the virus. The second mechanism is by the action of another viral protein, **B13R**. This protein acts intracellularly and blocks the activities of an enzyme, interleukin-1β-converting enzyme (ICE). ICE is important in the biosynthesis of IL-1β. However, this enzyme is also important in triggering apoptosis, and it is thought that blocking apoptosis is the more important function of vaccinia virus B13R.

The adenovirus (Ad) E1A protein (see section 3.2.2) blocks the transcription of the IL-6 gene, and it also interferes with the intracellular signalling cascade triggered by the binding of IL-6 to its cell-surface receptor. Ad also interferes with the cytolytic activities of TNF. This activity has been localized to the E3 region of the Ad genome because cells infected with wild-type Ad are resistant to TNF-induced lysis, while cells infected with mutant Ad lacking E3 are susceptible to lysis. Three products from E3 are responsible for resistance, although how these work is a mystery. These are the E3/10.4K, E3/14.5K and E3/14.7K proteins. The 14.7K protein is very abundant in the cytoplasm and nucleus of infected cells and is able to mediate resistance by itself. In contrast, the 10.4K and 14.5K proteins associate as a heterodimer in the plasma membrane of infected cells. In vaccinia virus there are two TNF-receptor homologues, A53R and B28R, although the genes are non-functional. Similar homologues have been located in variola virus and other animal poxviruses.

Some viruses interfere with the antiviral effects of interferons

The interferons (IFNs) are a family of related proteins that are grouped into three main species (α, β, γ) according to their functions and cellular source (reviewed by Landolfo *et al.*, 1995; Tyring, 1995; Jacobs and Langland, 1996). They were first discovered for their inhibitory effects on viral replication, although IFNs also influence a variety of other cellular activities. IFNs are released by cells that become infected by viruses, a process which is triggered by the presence of double-stranded RNA. Double-stranded RNA is not normally present in eukaryotic cells but it does appear in cells infected with many DNA viruses during the symmetrical transcription of their genomes. IFNs act in a paracrine fashion on uninfected cells close by and primes them to shut down protein synthesis should they subsequently become infected. There are over 14 different human IFN-α genes, whereas there are only single copies of IFN-β and IFN-γ genes. IFN-α and IFN-β (collectively termed type I interferons) are genetically related and produced by most cell types in response to virus infection. IFN-γ is unrelated to the type I interferons and is termed a type II interferon.

IFN-γ is produced by a limited number of lymphocytes (T_H1 cells, T_C cells and NK cells) and has many immunomodulatory properties in addition to antiviral activities.

The activities of IFN are mediated by binding to specific interferon receptors on cells. Both IFN-α and IFN-β bind to a common receptor, whereas IFN-γ binds to a separate receptor. Binding of IFN to a receptor leads to the activation of intracellular signalling pathways and induces the expression of at least 20 genes with a variety of antiviral and immunomodulatory effects. Several of the immunomodulatory properties were discussed in Chapter 1. In addition, IFNs signal cells to become more resistant to viral infection, mainly through inducing the expression of two important enzymes: **double-stranded**, **RNA-dependent**, **protein kinase** (or PKR), sometimes also called double-stranded, RNA-activated inhibitor (DAI), and **2′,5′-oligoadenylate synthase** (2,5-OS). Both of these enzymes are activated by double-stranded RNA.

The induction of PKR production by IFN results in the cell becoming poised to shut down protein synthesis should it become infected. PKR is normally inactive in uninfected cells, but becomes activated by autophosporylation in the presence of double-stranded RNA. When activated, PKR catalyses the phosphorylation of the α subunit of the translation initiating factor, eIF. eIF is an important component of the cellular protein-synthesis machinery, which is also required by many viruses for translation of their own RNA into viral protein. During translation of cellular mRNA into polypeptide, individual amino acids are delivered to the growing end of the polypeptide chain by tRNA. At each cycle, eIF is recycled by replacing GDP with GTP in a reaction catalysed by another enzyme, eIF-2B. When phosphorylated by PKR, eIF and eIF-2B form a tight complex which prevents eIF recycling and an abrupt halt to protein synthesis.

2′,5′-oligoadenylate synthase is also an interferon-inducible enzyme that is activated in the presence of double-stranded RNA. Its function is to polymerize ATP into oligomers of adenosines called oligoadenylate. The function of oligoadenylate is to activate an RNAase, that in turn rapidly degrades viral and cellular single-stranded RNA. Together, these two IFN-inducible pathways serve to cripple protein synthesis in the cell and prevent viral replication.

The importance of interferons in controlling viral infections is evident from the many viruses that possess countermeasures for interferons. Several viruses inhibit PKR by generating an abundance of non-coding, low-molecular-weight RNAs which serve as decoys for PKR. Such viruses include the human immunodeficiency virus (HIV), adenovirus (Ad) and Epstein–Barr virus (EBV). The Ad E1A protein also blocks IFN-induced gene expression by binding to a hitherto unidentified component of the IFN-induced intracellular signalling cascade. Other strategies include the synthesis of proteins by viruses that interfere with the products of IFN-inducible genes. For example, vaccinia virus produces two intracellular proteins, E3L and K3L. E3L blocks the activation of 2,5-OS and PKR by double-stranded RNA, and K3L blocks the autophosphorylation of eIF.

In addition to the intracellular mechanisms, vaccinia viruses are noted for producing an array of homologues of human cytokine receptors that are secreted from infected cells (reviewed by Alcami and Smith, 1995; Smith, 1996). Indeed, poxviruses appear to be the *only* group of viruses to express soluble cytokine receptors. Vaccinia's repertoire includes two soluble receptors for interferons: **B8R** which binds human IFN-γ, and **B18R** which binds IFN-α and IFN-β; and an abundant receptor for IL-1β called **B15R**. It has been noted that the affinities of these viral cytokine receptors vary between different strains of vaccinia. They appear to benefit the virus simply by neutralizing the biological activities of the cytokines and disrupting the cytokine network.

3.2.4 *Inhibition of complement*

Complement is one of the first host defence reactions encountered by invading viruses in the extracellular phase of their life cycle (see section 1.4.1 and review by Lachmann and Davies, 1997). Healthy cells in the body are protected from complement by a complex system of cell-surface and serum components that block various stages of the cascade. The γ-herpesvirus saimiri (HVS) has exploited these regulatory systems by capturing a number of genes that are homologous to human cellular counterparts including a homologue of decay-accelerating factor (DAF), and a protein that blocks activation of C9 and the assembly of the MAC.

Other herpesviruses, including HSV-1 and HSV-2, have a glycoprotein in their envelope called glycoprotein C (gC) that binds to the complement component C3b. The gC protein is also found in the plasma membrane of HSV-infected cells. The binding of C3b to gC fails to trigger the cascade, thereby providing an effective defence against complement although it is not known precisely how it works. A protein with a similar function, called glycoprotein III (gIII), is also found on pseudorabies virus, and on infected cells.

3.2.5 *Inhibition of apoptosis and inflammation*

Inflammation and apoptosis are the key antiviral responses that serve to limit the spread of infection. Inflammation, which is triggered by cell or tissue necrosis caused by viruses, is essential for exposing viral antigen to lymphocytes and for lymphocyte activation. Many viruses are lytic, thereby spilling their contents and causing inflammation. Cellular suicide by apoptosis is also an important, and phylogenetically ancient, antiviral defence mechanism. Apoptosis involves the activation of several 'suicide' genes which orchestrate first the fragmentation of DNA, followed by the systematic disruption of organelles, and finally the packaging of the digested cellular contents into non-inflammatory membrane-bound packages that are consumed by phagocytes. Not surprisingly, several viruses can interfere with inflammation and apoptosis in order to maintain the integrity of the host cell and thus to promote their own survival. Apoptosis is a large field and outside the scope of this book. The reader is referred to reviews for further information by Cuff and Ruby (1996) and Gillet and Brun (1996).

Summary of section 3.2

- Antigenic variation is employed by some viruses to escape from acquired immunity at both antibody and T-cell levels. Rhinovirus exists as over 160 serotypes (defined by neutralizing antibodies) with antigenically distinct capsid antigens that must all be encountered before full immunity is achieved. Influenza changes its surface antigens (mainly the haemagglutinin molecule) through the gradual accumulation of mutations (antigenic drift). Those that localize to surface epitopes lead to escape from pre-existing neutralizing antibody. Both rhinovirus and influenza are RNA viruses. Studies of EBV reveal that naturally occurring mutations might also allow escape from recognition by T_C cells.

- Several viruses escape recognition by T_C cells by producing proteins that block the class I MHC antigen-processing pathway at strategic points. Notable are adenovirus E3/19K that arrests class I heavy chains in the ER, herpes simplex virus ICP47 that blocks transport of peptides through the TAP1/TAP2 transporter, and the gp24 protein of cytomegalovirus that dislocates nascent class I heavy chains from the ER back into the cytosol where they are degraded by the proteasome. CMV also produces a homologue of the class I heavy chain, that leads to surface expression of a non-functional heterodimer with β_2m; this is thought to block NK lysis.

- Other viruses interfere with the cytokine network. Of interest is the Epstein–Barr virus homologue of IL-10 which down-regulates the antiviral effects of T_H1 cells and promotes B-cell proliferation as a source of new host cells. Poxviruses produce an array of soluble cytokine receptors which are thought to disrupt the delicate balance of the cytokine milieu. Among these are soluble IFN receptors which may block their antiviral effects by binding extracellularly. Other viruses interfere with IFNs intracellularly – HIV and adenovirus produce small RNA molecules to prevent the activation of double-stranded, RNA-dependent, protein kinase which shuts down protein synthesis in response to double-stranded viral RNA.

- Many other mechanisms exist, including interference with complement, apoptosis and inflammation, and others not discussed here, such as chemokines, tyrosine kineases involved in signalling cascades, and so on. Others are no doubt waiting to be discovered.

Study problems for section 3.2

1. Give evidence for how antigenic variation enables viruses to evade cell-mediated and antibody-mediated immunity.
2. Give examples of viral homologues of human cytokines or cytokine receptors and suggest how they may be beneficial to the virus.
3. What are the antiviral activities of complement and how do some viruses counteract complement.

3.3 Influenza virus

Despite the many advances in the scientific understanding of infectious diseases, influenza remains an enigma and attempts to control the viruses that cause the disease appear to have failed. The fascination with influenza is partly due to the history of the great pandemics and the worldwide devastation these outbreaks have caused, and partly due to the panic an outbreak of a new strain of influenza invokes amongst the tabloid press. The major pandemics of influenza A viruses over the last hundred years are shown in Table 3.5. Of particular note is the 1918–1919 pandemic, which is believed to have resulted in more deaths in 9–12 months than occurred through the mighty battles of the Great War. Part of the fascination with the 1918 pandemic was

Table 3.5 The major influenza A pandemics

Era	Approximate periods	Subtype
H2-H3N2 era	1889–1890	H2N2
	1900	H3N2
Swine era	1918–1919	Swine-like virus
	1934, 1946	H1N1
H3N2 era	1957–1958	H2N2
	1968	H3N2

that, unusually, deaths occurred predominantly amongst the 15 to 50 year age group. The potential for such destruction amongst this age group has invoked much discussion amongst novelists and the many prophets of doom writing popular science books.

Influenza was first suspected of being a virus in 1933 when Smith, Andrewes and Laidlaw found that transmission was mediated by a filterable agent. In 1941, Hirst and McCleland discovered that influenza viruses haemagglutinated chick red blood cells and this was to form the basis of the haemagglutination and the complementary haemagglutination inhibition test that is still important in the research of influenza viruses. The subsequent discovery that influenza viruses grew in embryonated hens eggs enabled the growth of high titres of purified virus and facilitated the molecular understanding of how this virus causes disease. Of major interest in this family of viruses is the frequent emergence of novel antigenic variants as the source of pandemics, and the analysis of the mechanisms responsible.

The impact of any virus on a population reflects a combination of the prevalence of infection and the severity of the disease inflicted. Prevalence is due to the ease by which the virus can spread through a susceptible population, whereas severity may be determined by the ability of the virus to cause tissue damage directly. Influenza causes epidemics both in man and in many species of mammals and birds and the latter offer a substantial reservoir of the viruses that as yet have not crossed the species barrier and infected man. At the time of writing (early 1998) much attention is being focused on an H5N1 strain of influenza A virus that has so far infected 14 individuals in Hong Kong with four deaths. A lot of resources are being committed to contain this new human strain, including the culling of over one million domestic chickens which are thought to be the main reservoir for the virus. Already, researchers are busy developing a vaccine just in case the virus escapes attempts to contain it.

Whatever the outcome of the new epidemic, there can be little doubt that this virus demands the utmost respect and outbreaks of new strains in humans will continue to evoke panic.

3.3.1 *Pathogenesis*

Influenza spreads from person to person by airborne droplets or contact with contaminated hands or surfaces. A few cells of respiratory epithelium are infected if deposited virus particles avoid removal by respiratory cilia, the cough reflex, and escape neutralization by pre-existing IgA antibodies or by non-specific inhibitors in mucous membranes. Replication is rapid. Progeny virions are produced as early as 6 h after infection and spread to adjacent epithelial cells, where the replication cycle is repeated. The viral neuraminidase aids in cell-to-cell transmission by lowering the viscosity of the mucous film in the respiratory tract to facilitate the attachment of virus to receptors on the surface of underlying epithelial cells.

The rapidity of replication leads to an incubation period from time of exposure to symptoms of 1–4 days, depending partly on the initial dose of the virus and on the immunocompetence of the host. The shedding of virus begins before the onset of symptoms and peaks 1–2 days after the onset of symptoms, after which shedding declines rapidly. Interferons are detectable in respiratory secretions 1 day after the detection of virus shedding and represent one of the earliest immunological responses to the virus infection. In contrast, specific antibodies and T_C cells cannot be detected for 7–14 days. T_C cells play a vital role in eliminating the infection, while antibodies serve to block any future re-infection by the same subtype of virus. Indeed it was studies with influenza nucleoprotein (NP)-specific T_C cells that led to the breakthroughs in understanding the class I MHC antigen-processing pathway (reviewed by Townsend and Bodmer, 1989; Parker and Gould, 1996).

Inflammation of the upper respiratory tract causes necrosis of the ciliated epithelium of both the trachea and bronchi which takes approximately 4 weeks to repair. Influenza virus destruction of the respiratory tract lowers the host's resistance to secondary bacterial infection. Bronchial pneumonia caused by *Staphylococcus aureus*, *Streptococcus pneumoniae* or *Haemophilus influenzae* remain a major complication and cause of death in influenza virus-induced disease. Symptoms of influenza appear abruptly and include chills, headache, muscle aches and high fever which lasts 3 or more days.

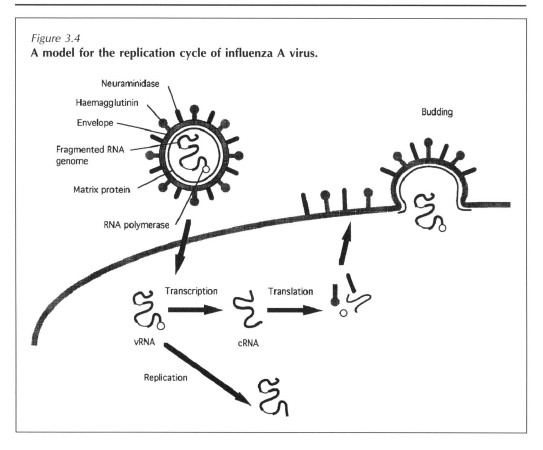

Figure 3.4
A model for the replication cycle of influenza A virus.

3.3.2 *Replication of influenza viruses*

Influenzas are pleomorphic, enveloped viruses approximately 100 nm in diameter. The genome is negative-sense single-stranded RNA, which is divided into eight separate segments. Most of the segments encode a single protein, and the presence of two different influenza A viruses within the same cell can give rise to exchange of segments called **genetic reassortment**.

Two antigens on the surface of the envelope, haemagglutinin (HA) and neuraminidase (NA), are important in antigenic diversity of the virus. The virus HA molecule is composed of two chains, HA1 and HA2. HA1 forms a globular head to the molecule which mediates attachment of the virus to sialic acid residues on the host cell membrane. HA2 connects the globular head to the envelope of the virus, and also mediates fusion of the envelope with the cell plasma membrane. This is accompanied by the proteolytic cleavage of HA2, which is a pH-dependent process. The viral RNA is then released into the cell cytoplasm (Figure 3.4).

Transcription of viral RNA differs to that of other RNA viruses in that cellular functions are essential and that viral

RNA is transcribed in the nucleus of the host cell. The virus-encoded RNA polymerase is primarily responsible for viral RNA transcription but requires help in priming from cellular RNA polymerase II. Viral genome replication is achieved by the same enzymes involved in transcription. The mechanism by which the various influenza genome segments are assembled into progeny virions is not known. The virus matures by budding from the host cell membrane. Replication is quite rapid, with progeny viruses detectable from 6 to 8 h after infection. As many as 90 per cent of progeny virions are defective and therefore non-infectious.

3.3.3 *Pandemic influenza infections are associated with antigenic shift*

There are three major serotypes of influenza A, namely A, B and C. These are classified according to the antigenicity of the HA and NA molecules. Of these there are several subtypes. When one includes the influenza viruses of mammals (in particular, horses, pigs and man) and birds, there are in all 14 HA subtypes (H1, H2, H3, etc.) and 9 NA subtypes (N1, N2, N3, etc.). Reassortment is thought to occur between HA and NA gene segments of human influenza A virus with a virus from another species during co-infection in a single mammalian or avian host. This leads to sudden changes in the surface HA and NA molecules from one subtype to another, a process called **antigenic shift**.

The introduction of new influenza A subtypes into man results in worldwide outbreaks or **pandemics**. Since the influenza pandemic of 1918, there have been pandemics in 1934, 1946, 1957 and 1968. The fact that only three HA and three NA subtypes have infected humans leaves ample opportunity for pandemics to emerge with other HA and NA subtypes. Influenza A was first isolated in 1933 and this virus was designated H1N1. The 1957 pandemic was caused by a shift in the HA and NA genes resulting in the H2N2 subtype, whilst the 1968 pandemic was caused by the H3N2 subtype. In between pandemics, **epidemics** occur almost annually (see below).

Each pandemic occurs because antibodies to each subtype provide only weak neutralization of other subtypes. For example, serum obtained from a subject infected with an H1N1 virus (strain A/PR/8/34) is capable of neutralizing the homologous H1N1 virus, even after dilution. However, this serum offers no protection against the 1946 H1N1 virus or the subsequent 1957 H2N2 or 1968 H3N2 viruses. Therefore, any individual previously infected with H1N1 virus is totally susceptible to infection with any H2N2 or H3N2 virus.

Molecular analyses of the HA and NA genes have revealed a high degree of sequence diversity between different subtypes. The amino acid sequence homology between H1 and H3 is 35 per cent, and between H2 and H3 is 40 per cent, whereas the homology between H1 and H2 is more conserved at 70 per cent. Similarly, the amino acid sequence homology between N1 and N2 is around 41 per cent. This degree of variation results in viruses that are unaffected by antibodies directed against the glycoproteins of other virus subtypes. This enables the newly mutated subtype to replicate unchecked in susceptible hosts.

Prior to the introduction of the H3N2 virus into humans, examples of H3 viruses had been isolated from birds and horses, as for example in A/Duck/Ukraine/1/63/H3N8 and A/Equine/Miami/1/63/H3N8. It is considered highly likely that the human H3 subtype virus arose by recombination between a human virus and an animal influenza virus to produce a virus with pathogenic potential for man. In this instance the HA gene was thought to have arisen from an avian host because homology between the H3 gene of the human and avian strains is around 90 per cent, whilst the homology between the human and equine strains is approximately 80 per cent. Therefore, the 1968 pandemic was caused by the introduction of a novel HA into a non-immune population.

3.3.4 *Epidemics are associated with antigenic drift*

The ability of influenza A subtypes to persist and cause epidemic disease in the population is thought to be due to a different process. The replication of RNA viruses is very inefficient and this causes point mutations and an accumulation of amino acid substitutions in the viral antigens. In influenza, mutations in the HA and NA glycoproteins can lead to changes in the epitopes recognized by neutralizing antibodies. This gradual accumulation of amino acid changes is known as **antigenic drift**, and is different to antigenic shift in which wholesale exchange of genetic information occurs. Antigenic drift in the influenza HA and NA antigens leads to regular epidemics because novel viruses escape elimination by the neutralizing antibodies raised to previously encountered strains. Drift may contribute to escape from memory T lymphocytes as well.

Comparisons have been made between the nucleotide sequences of the HA and NA genes from influenza strains

Figure 3.5

Natural variation between influenza haemagglutinin molecules localizes to five distinct sites that correspond to surface epitopes recognized by neutralizing antibodies (see Wiley et al., 1981).

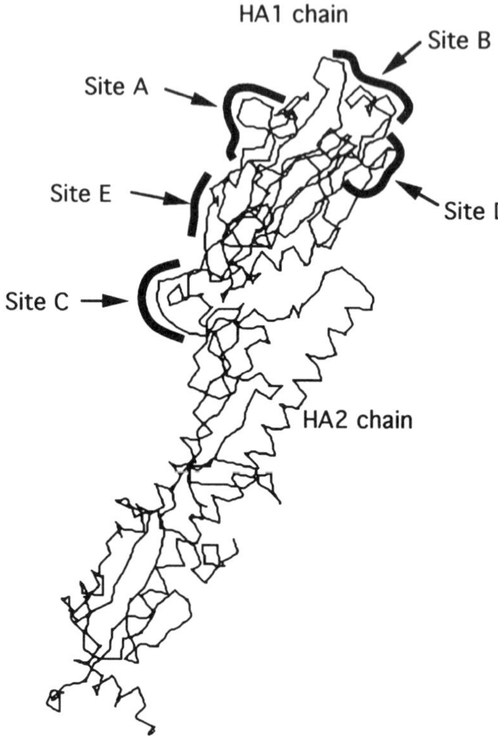

isolated during different epidemics. The amino acid changes that accompanied each epidemic could then be identified. These data have been supplemented with sequences from laboratory-generated escape mutants that were selected on the basis of being able to overcome neutralization by HA-specific monoclonal antibodies. When these amino acid changes are mapped to the three-dimensional structure of the HA molecule obtained by X-ray crystallography, it can be seen that they cluster into distinct surface-located regions. Each corresponds to an epitope recognized by a neutralizing antibody. In this way, five epitopes have been mapped on the molecule (Figure 3.5). The emergence of each epidemiologically significant strain of influenza A requires amino acid substitutions in at least three of the different neutralizing epitopes on HA.

In summary, antigenic shift is characterized by large sudden changes in the HA or NA genes, probably due to recombination of a human virus with a virus from another species. In contrast, antigenic drift is characterized by a constant change in the HA and NA proteins driven by immunological escape mutants. Mutations in at least three antibody epitopes of HA are required for an epidemiologically important strain to emerge.

3.3.5 *Pathogenicity*

The pathogenicity of a virus should always be considered in relation to the host. In nature the creation of a pathogenic influenza A virus occurred in the winter of 1979–1980 when many dead seals were found on the New England coast of the USA. From the lungs and brains of these dead animals, an influenza A virus was isolated which was found to be a reassortment of two known Asian viruses not previously known to infect seals. It is by no means an advantage for a virus to be highly pathogenic because the virus may inadvertently eradicate susceptible hosts.

Human H3N2 viruses cannot be transmitted directly to birds without reassortment in pigs. Species specificity is apparently determined by the NA protein. Pigs are likely hosts in which mixing between strains may occur to cause antigenic shift and the start of new pandemics. Agricultural practices in South-East Asia, where pigs, ducks and humans may live in close proximity, may facilitate this process.

3.3.6 *Prevention and treatment*

Two drugs are available for the treatment of influenza: amantidine and rimantidine. These compounds work by preventing the uncoating of the virus. This is achieved by blocking the passage of protons through the viral matrix protein that is required for the pH-dependent changes in the haemagglutinin protein which lead to uncoating. These drugs are reported to be approximately 70 per cent effective in protecting against subsequent infection with influenza A. Other compounds are under investigation. In particular, one very promising compound from Glaxo Wellcome is currently in clinical trials (zanamivir) and is an analogue of the viral neuraminidase. In addition there are a number of inactivated vaccines available for the protection of individuals against influenza A. However, existing vaccines are being constantly rendered ineffective due to the constant mutation of circulating strains.

Summary of section 3.3

- Influenza A viruses have long been associated with large worldwide outbreaks of disease known as pandemics. In between the pandemics the virus is able to sustain itself in human populations in smaller epidemics. The molecular basis for these outbreaks is derived from changes in the external envelope proteins, haemagglutinin (HA) and neuraminidase (NA). Changes in the hypervariable regions within the surface component of the HA1 subunit result in viral escape from neutralizing antibody. Variation in other antigens such as nucleoprotein (NP) may aid escape from T_C cells.

- The process by which influenza viruses are able to escape immune detection is dependent on the gradual accumulation of spontaneous mutations in major antigens (antigenic drift). This enables the virus to establish epidemics within a partially susceptible community. The segmented nature of the virus genome allows reassortment to occur between two viruses with different HA molecules, for example, when an H2N2 virus recombines with an H3N1 virus to produce H2N1 or H3N2 progeny (antigenic shift). These may represent a new subtype of influenza which has not previously been experienced by the host, resulting in pandemics.

Study problems for section 3.3

1. What are the mechanisms by which influenza A viruses cause epidemics and pandemics in humans?
2. What are the key features of the replication cycle of influenza viruses that allow for new strains of the virus to emerge?
3. What are the main difficulties that need to be overcome in order to develop an effective vaccine against all strains of influenza?

3.4   The human immunodeficiency virus

The human immunodeficiency virus is the cause of the **acquired immunodeficiency syndrome** (AIDS), which first came to prominence in the early 1980s when previously healthy homosexual men came down with overwhelming immunodeficiencies. The early cases of AIDS reported in 1981 presented with *Pneumocystis carinii* pneumonia (PCP) or Kaposi's sarcoma, a previously rare form of skin cancer. Close investigation of the early cases of AIDS showed a large reduction in CD4-bearing T-helper lymphocytes from approximately 1000 cells per µl of blood to undetectable levels in some patients. From the very beginning of the epidemic a viral infection was suspected as the likely cause. In 1983, scientists at the Pasteur Institute in Paris were the first to isolate a retrovirus from an individual with immunodeficiency and the virus was given the name lymphadenopathy-associated virus (LAV). American scientists subsequently confirmed that a retrovirus was responsible for causing the immunodeficiency that led to AIDS but named the virus either human T-lymphotropic virus type III (HTLV-III) or AIDS-related virus (ARV). In 1986 the virus was renamed human immunodeficiency virus (HIV). Not everyone believes that HIV is the cause of AIDS and much controversy has surrounded the syndrome and the viruses that cause it. In 1986, scientists at the Pasteur Institute in Paris discovered a second virus in patients with AIDS in West Africa and this virus was named HIV-2. The discovery of AIDS-like viruses from several different species of monkeys led to the hypothesis that HIV originated in monkeys and at some point relatively recently crossed the species barrier to infect man.

Since the discovery of HIV, the virus has been subjected to intense research in order to find a cure for the disease. Already there are an estimated 14 million cases of AIDS worldwide and the World Health Organization predicts that this may rise to 40 million by the year 2000. HIV-1 is the predominant cause of AIDS worldwide and has infected over 1 million individuals in North America, over 500 000 in Western Europe, and approximately 15 000 in Australia. In these countries homosexual men account for about 60 per cent of all cases, 25 per cent occurring in intravenous drug users and the remaining 15 per cent spread between the heterosexual community and other high-risk groups such as haemophiliacs. In sub-Saharan Africa, South America, India and South-East Asia the virus is sexually transmitted and it is found in equal frequency in men and women.

Despite intense research there is still no vaccine. In the Western world HIV is held in check by a combination of antiretroviral drugs, but despite powerful combinations of compounds, many individuals still progress to AIDS and death.

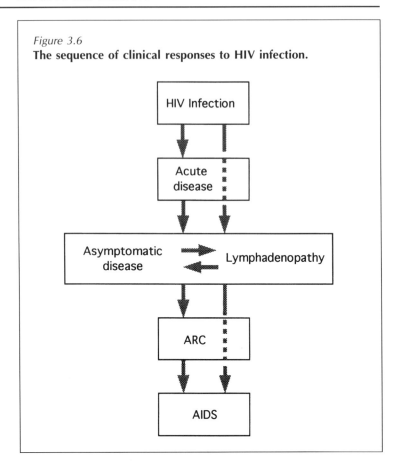

Figure 3.6
The sequence of clinical responses to HIV infection.

3.4.1 *Pathogenesis*

The various stages of HIV-1 infection leading to AIDS are summarized in Figure 3.6. Transmission of HIV-1 may be through homosexual or heterosexual contact as extracellular virus in semen or vaginal secretions, or within infected leucocytes such as CD4+ T lymphocytes or macrophages. Transmission may also occur through contact with contaminated blood products during transfusion, intravenous drug abuse, or by laboratory needlestick injury.

Following exposure, one of two things may occur. First, no infection may occur, and several studies have placed the likelihood of transmission of the virus from 0.5 to 10 per cent for a single exposure episode. Recently, a number of studies have shown that patients who have a deletion in the second HIV-1 receptor protein CC-R5 have a reduced risk of transmission of the virus. Normally, CC-R5 is the cellular receptor on the surface of peripheral blood mononuclear cells for the β-**chemokines** RANTES, MIP-1α and MIP-1β (Box 3.1).

These are cytokines that have chemotactic properties for blood mononuclear cells. High levels of these chemokines circulating in peripheral blood are known to protect against HIV infection by saturating all available receptor sites. The alternative consequence of exposure is infection. Primary infection of host CD4+ cells (T cells and dendritic cells) usually occurs in lymph nodes draining the site of entry wherein the virus replicates. The virus is disseminated from these sites of replication and high levels of blood-borne virus (viraemia) ensue. The level of virus replication at this stage of infection may well be a prognostic factor in the speed at which the patient proceeds to AIDS. Accompanying the viraemia, the patient may experience primary disease symptoms (called seroconversion illness) including a generalized maculopapular rash, pneumonitis, and gastrointestinal and brain involvement.

Box 3.1 **Chemokines**

Chemokines are a large group of cytokines that are generated during inflamation. As the name suggests, these cytokines have chemotactic properties and act as chemical attractants for cells with chemokine receptors. Chemokines are classified into α- and β-chemokines according to function and sequence homology: the α-chemokines have a characteristic cys–x–cys motif (CXC) and attract mainly neutrophils, whereas β-chemokines have a charcteristic cys–cys motif (CC) and attract mainly monocytes and lymphocytes. A common feature of chemokines is that their receptors are all members of the superfamily of G-protein linked receptors. These are so called because in response to binding an extracellular ligand, their cytoplasmic domains become associated with a GTP-binding protein (G-protein). G-protein linked receptors all have a distinctive seven-span transmembrane domain.

Recently, chemokine receptors have been found to be important second receptors in HIV infection (see table). These include CC-R5 and CXC-4. CC-R5 is the natural receptor on peripheral blood mononuclear cells for the β-chemokines RANTES, MIP-1α and MIP-1β. CXC-4 is the receptor on T cells whose ligands include IL-8. IL-8 is a cytokine with chemotactic and activation properties for neutrophils. The role of this cytokine could also be important in HIV-1 infected patients with *Pneumocystis carinii* pneumonia because there is a direct correlation between neutrophil infiltration into the lung and severity of disease. MIP-1 is a chemoattractant for CD8+ T_C cells and activates neutrophils and monocytes.

Chemokine receptors associated with HIV-1 entry into cells

Chemokine receptor	Family	Natural ligand
CXC-4	α	IL-8, GRO-α, NAP-2
CC-R3	β	Eotaxin, RANTES, MCP-3
CC-R5	β	MIP-1α, MIP-1β, RANTES

During this initial period of infection the virus is disseminated to other lymph nodes via trafficking T cells. The patient then progresses to the second stage of HIV disease, termed progressive generalized lymphadenopathy. This is characterized by lymph node swelling (lymphadenopathy) which is indicative of an active immune response to the virus. At this point in the infection the first antibodies emerge (seroconversion) and may reach high levels. Moreover, a strong CD8+ T_C cell is generated which results in the clearance of HIV from the blood. This is an asymptomatic 'clinically latent' phase of the disease which may last for years. During this period the virus is confined mainly to the lymph nodes where approximately 10^9 new virus particles are made every day.

Infection of CD4+ T cells and the production of new virions causes T-cell death. The rate at which new virions are produced is in dynamic contrast to the rate of production of new CD4+ T cells in the bone marrow each day to compensate. The half-life of HIV in plasma is approximately 10 min, whereas in newly infected CD4+ T cells it is about 2.5 days. That is, each productively infected CD4+ cell is replaced every 5 days. Approximately, 98 per cent of HIV-infected cells are productively infected CD4+ lymphocytes, about 1 per cent are latently infected T-lymphocytes and the remaining 1 per cent are chronically infected macrophages and dendritic cells (Figure 3.7). Additional information about the dynamics of viral replication can be found in Coffin (1995), Ho *et al.* (1995), Wei *et al.* (1995) and Perelson *et al.* (1997).

The third phase of HIV disease is reached when the number of CD4+ T cells in the blood (which is normally 1000 per μl) falls to 200–500 cells per μl. This stage, which was originally termed **AIDS related complex** (ARC), is characterized by non-specific indications of immunosuppression that include *Candida* infections such as oral and vaginal thrush, and reactivation of herpesvirus infections such as cold sores, genital herpes and shingles. Reactivation of tuberculosis is a complication which may occur during this phase of the illness and this particular manifestation is now classified as a diagnostic symptom of full-blown AIDS. Tuberculosis is a particularly serious complication as the prevalence of multiple drug-resistant (MDR) strains of *Mycobacterium tuberculosis* necessitates both short-course treatment lasting 6 months and longer-term treatment lasting a year.

During this terminal phase of disease, HIV is actively replicating in the lymph nodes of the infected individuals and the plasma levels of virus may be quite low or even

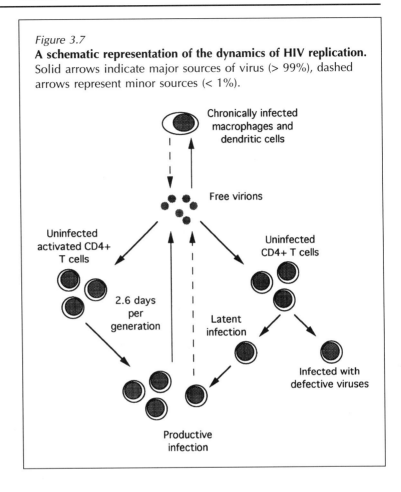

Figure 3.7
A schematic representation of the dynamics of HIV replication.
Solid arrows indicate major sources of virus (> 99%), dashed
arrows represent minor sources (< 1%).

below the cut-off of the assays (less than 400 copies of HIV
RNA/ml of plasma). Disagreement exists as to how HIV-
infected patients in this stage of disease should be managed.
In particular, whether all patients should be given triple
combination antiretroviral therapy in an attempt to eliminate the virus, or whether to only treat patients who have a
viral load of greater than 30 000 copies per ml of plasma.
However, all patients who are progressing to AIDS, as measured by rapidly falling CD4+ cell counts, will probably start
therapy.

The fourth stage of the disease is defined as full-blown
AIDS and is reached usually when the patient's CD4+ cell
count has dropped to below 200 cells per μl of blood.
AIDS-defining illnesses include infection with a number of
opportunistic diseases including *Pneumocystis carinii* pneumonia (PCP), *Cryptosporidium* infections, toxoplasmosis,
retinitis caused by cytomegalovirus, and diseases caused by
the *Mycobacterium intracellulare–avium* complex. AIDS may

also be defined in patients who develop unusual forms of cancer such as Kaposi's sarcoma, which is now believed to be caused by human herpesvirus type 8 (HHV8). Non-Hodgkin's lymphomas may also develop during this stage of disease. Other life-threatening diseases such as various types of bacterial pneumonias and gastrointestinal parasitic infections associated with severe weight loss become more common.

During AIDS, HIV levels in the blood increase dramatically due to the destruction of the germinal centres of the lymph nodes. The biological characteristics of the virus recovered from the blood may also change. Prior to AIDS, the viruses are slow-growing, non-cytopathic (**non-syncytium inducing** or NSI) strains that only grow in primary cell lines such as macrophages. After the onset of AIDS, they are more pathogenic, rapidly replicating viruses that are highly cytopathic and cause cell fusion *in vitro* (called **syncytium inducing** or SI strains). These will grow to very high titre in established T-cell lines *in vitro*. The average length of time from primary HIV infection to development of full-blown AIDS is 10 years, whilst the average time from full-blown AIDS to death is 17 months.

3.4.2 *Replication of human immunodeficiency virus*

The replication of HIV is probably the best understood of all viruses (see Greene, 1991). A schematic diagram of the HIV genome structure is shown in Figure 3.8. The virus consists of a long terminal repeat (LTR) at the 5′ end of the genome which contains the promoter, enhancer and host cell DNA-binding protein domains. Downstream of the LTR are three major coding regions. The *gag* gene encodes the structural proteins, including the p24 antigen that forms the major capsid protein. Antibodies to this antigen form the basis of the HIV test. Next is the polymerase (*pol*) gene which contains the viral protease, reverse transcriptase, RNAaseH and integrase enzymes. The next gene is the envelope (*env*) gene which includes the gp120 and gp41 proteins; these form the CD4-binding proteins and envelope fusion protein, respectively. At the 3′ end of the genome is an LTR and this enables the viral genome to link with the 5′ LTR and form a circular plasmid-type structure.

In addition to these three major reading frames (which are found in all exogenous retroviruses), HIV contains a number of accessory genes, some of which are essential for replication. The transcription of transactivation (*tat*) gene

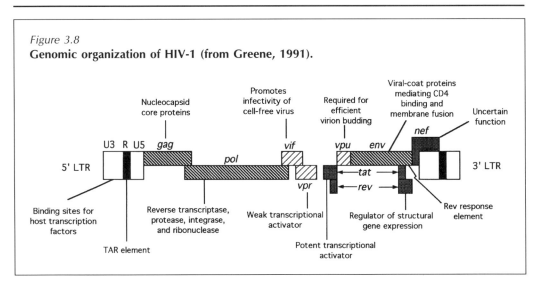

Figure 3.8
Genomic organization of HIV-1 (from Greene, 1991).

encodes a protein that is essential for the replication of HIV. Tat is produced in abundance early in the replication of the virus. The product of the ***rev*** gene is a regulator of structural gene expression and is also essential for the replication of the virus. The rev protein enables the completion of HIV replication by enabling full-length RNA to be transported to the cytoplasm to enable the transcription of full-length structural proteins which are then transported to the cell surface for assembly. Full genomic RNA is also required for the completion of infectious progeny virions. The replication of HIV is very inefficient and the ratio of non-infectious, defective, viral particles to infectious viral particles is 10 000 to 1. Other viral genes include ***vpr*** which encodes a weak transcriptional factor, ***vif*** which encodes a viral infectivity factor, ***vpu*** which is required for efficient virion budding, and ***nef*** which has an uncertain function.

Attachment

HIV is an enveloped virus, approximately 100 nm in diameter, containing two copies of positive-sense, single-stranded RNA. The replication cycle of HIV is depicted in Figure 3.9. The virus attaches to the CD4 molecule on the surface of susceptible cells, although there are some reports of CD4-independent infection of some cell types. Before the virus can gain entry into the cell it must attach to a second receptor on the surface of the host cell. Attachment to the second receptor is via the third hypervariable region of the gp120 protein on the surface of the virus, the so-called V3 loop. Two second receptors have been discovered, CC-R5 and

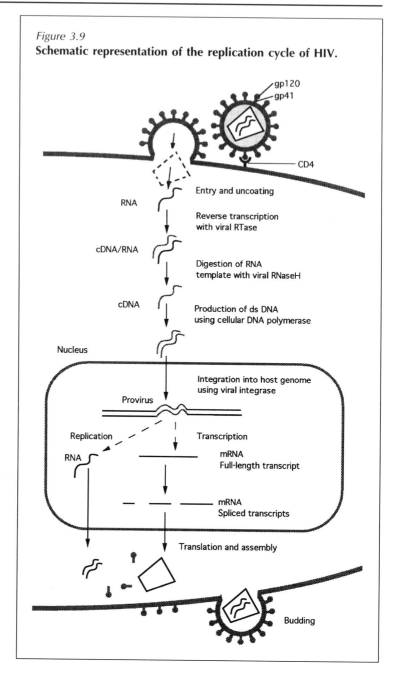

Figure 3.9
Schematic representation of the replication cycle of HIV.

CXC-4, which as mentioned earlier are normally chemokine receptors (Box 3.1). Usage of one or other of these second receptors is important in distinguishing the biological characteristics of the HIV strain. CC-R5 is used by slow-growing, NSI macrophage strains of HIV and the receptor is found mainly on the surface of monocytes and macrophages. CXC-4 is found on the surface of T lymphocytes and also on established T-cell lines and is the second receptor for the rapidly-growing SI strains of HIV.

Entry and transcription

Following attachment of gp120 to the second receptor, the protein is cleaved by host cell proteases. The viral envelope then fuses with the surface of the host cell via the N-terminal gp41 transmembrane protein that contains a fusion domain. Once the virus has entered the cell the capsid is broken down, releasing the viral RNA into the cytoplasm of the cell. Reverse transcriptase present in the infecting viral particle transcribes the viral RNA to DNA. The RNA–DNA hybrid is broken down by viral RNAaseH and the second strand of viral DNA is completed by the reverse transcriptase enzyme. The double-stranded DNA molecule is transported to the nucleus of the cell where it is integrated into the host cell chromosome. At this point, HIV may remain latent (that is, transcriptionally inactive) until the T cell is activated in response to antigen.

During the replication of the virus, both spliced RNA transcripts and full-length RNA species are transported to the ribosomes in the cytoplasm for translation. The viral proteins and full-length genomic RNA are transported to the cell membrane for assembly of the virus. HIV obtains an envelope by budding through the host cell membrane; the envelope is made up of 80 per cent of host cell membrane but also contains the viral transmembrane protein gp41 and the viral extracellular protein gp120.

Dynamics of HIV replication

It has now become clear that the level of HIV replication within individuals is very important in the rate of progression to AIDS and death. As illustrated in Figure 3.10, there is a statistically significant relationship between HIV load in plasma (as determined by viral RNA) and progression to AIDS. Patients with a viral load of less than 4530 copies per ml progressed to AIDS at a statistically significant slower rate than patients who had a viral load of between 4531 and 13 020 copies per ml (Mellors *et al.*, 1996). The biggest difference in progression to AIDS was between those with a viral load of less than 4530 copies and those with a viral load of more than 36 270 copies per ml.

As shown in Figure 3.7, HIV in actively replicating T cells is replaced every 2.6 days. By applying strong drug

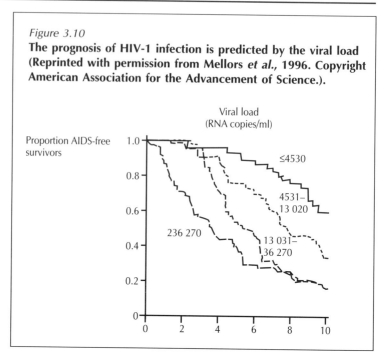

Figure 3.10

The prognosis of HIV-1 infection is predicted by the viral load (Reprinted with permission from Mellors *et al.*, 1996. Copyright American Association for the Advancement of Science.).

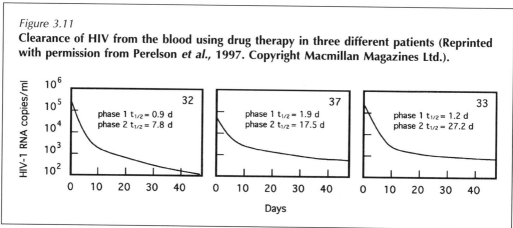

Figure 3.11

Clearance of HIV from the blood using drug therapy in three different patients (Reprinted with permission from Perelson *et al.*, 1997. Copyright Macmillan Magazines Ltd.).

pressure to a completely sensitive virus it has been possible to monitor the clearance of HIV from the blood. The clearance is biphasic (Figure 3.11). Initially, HIV is cleared from productively infected cells with a half-life of less than 2 days, followed by phase 2 clearance from latently or chronically infected cells that can take as long as 28 days. Extrapolating these data it is possible to predict that to eliminate the virus entirely from the host would take 3.1 years of total suppression of virus from plasma. To suppress HIV replication sufficiently for its elimination, it is necessary to initiate infected patients on at least triple combination antiretroviral therapy. A combination of **nucleoside analogues** (such as AZT, 3TC, ddI, ddC, D4T or 1592U) and **protease inhibitors** (such as saquinavir, indinavir, ritonavir, nelfinavir or 141W) are commonly used. Further treatment options include the non-nucleoside inhibitors such as nevirapine or delavirdine. First-line treatment options usually involve two nucleoside analogues and a protease inhibitor and favourite combinations include AZT, 3TC plus indinavir or ddI, D4T plus ritonavir.

3.4.3 *Immunological escape by HIV*

Within 4 to 8 weeks of HIV infection the host produces a strong T_C-cell response which coincides with a reduction in virus levels in plasma. The host also produces antibodies against a number of HIV proteins, notably p24, gp120 and gp41 envelope proteins. Within the gp120 protein the major neutralizing epitope is located within the V3 loop. As a consequence of neutralizing antibodies, immunological pressure is applied to the virus and replication is halted unless the virus mutates and escapes neutralization by antibodies (or detection by T_C-cell).

One of the major problems in controlling the progression of HIV disease is that codon changes occur (on average once per replication cycle) due to the infidelity of reverse transcriptase and the lack of viral correction enzymes. If the codon change results in a stop codon being inserted into the middle of a viral protein, the mutation is lethal to replication and a defective virus particle is produced. Alternatively, in the case of a mutation in a viral enzyme, such as the protease gene, viral replication cannot be completed.

Certain regions of the viral genome, called **hypervariable regions** are more prone to mutations. These occur particularly in the *env*-encoded proteins. For example, there are five such regions in gp120, termed V1 toV5. It is mutations in this protein which enable the virus to escape antibody neutralization and to continue replication. The V3 loop appears to be particularly important in this respect. Prior to the development of antibodies to HIV, the circulating virus is quite homologous; it is the application of immunological pressure which results in viral variants. In short, the immune system drives the diversity of the virus. Indeed, it has been calculated that due to the dynamic rate of HIV replication *in vivo*, every available single-point mutation is in place before antiretroviral therapy is normally initiated.

The reason that the virus appears homologous prior to the immune response may be due to the growth advantage

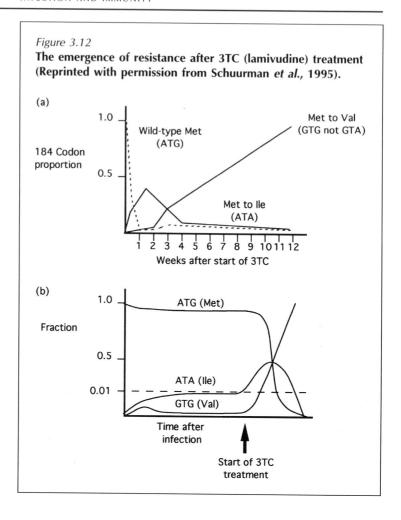

Figure 3.12

The emergence of resistance after 3TC (lamivudine) treatment (Reprinted with permission from Schuurman *et al.*, 1995).

the wild-type virus has over the mutants. This has been well described for HIV mutants that show increased resistance to antiretroviral agents, as is illustrated in Figure 3.12 for lamivudine (3TC) treatment. One point mutation in the reverse transcriptase gene at position 184 from methionine to valine results in a 100- to 1000-fold increase in resistance to 3TC. If a patient is placed on 3TC monotherapy, the wild-type virus, which has a distinct growth advantage over the mutant, is quickly eliminated from the plasma and is replaced within 4 weeks by the mutant virus. However, if the drug is withdrawn, the wild-type virus quickly returns.

3.4.4 *Development of an HIV vaccine*

Several approaches have been made to develop an effective vaccine to HIV. A recent perspective is given by Burton

(1997). These approaches include whole virus vaccines from live attenuated virus, formalin-fixed virus, and viruses which are defective. Subunit vaccines based on gp160, gp120 and gp41 proteins expressed in bacteria, animal cells or as part of the external proteins of virus vectors, have been produced. Each of these approaches has inherent problems associated with it. In general, an effective vaccine needs to protect against all the HIV strains in circulation. However, this is a formidable problem for several reasons. The antigenic drift of the virus and recombination between strains ensures continuing evolution and escape. Moreover, an effective vaccine has to protect against the mucosal spread of the virus, as well as transmission via infected cells and by cell fusion. HIV also establishes a life-long latent infection of some cell types without revealing its presence to T cells. Finally, HIV infects and destroys several cells central to the well-being of the adaptive immune system. The development of a vaccine against HIV remains a big challenge.

Summary of section 3.4

- HIV is a retrovirus that is the causative agent of AIDS. The low fidelity of viral enzymes involved in replication enables the virus to mutate readily and as a consequence escape an adaptive immune response. The virus readily compromises the immune system because it infects and replicates in the very cells of the immune system that are required to effect its removal. The dynamics of HIV replication are such that the half-life of the virus in plasma is approximately 6 h, and the half-life in actively replicating CD4+ T cells is 2.5 days. Therefore, the replication of the virus in the host is a dynamic process, with the virus being predominantly centralized in the lymph nodes early in infection, but erupting into the circulation late in the course of the disease.

Study problems for section 3.4

1. What obstacles still remain before a safe and effective HIV vaccine will be available?
2. How does an intricate knowledge of the replication cycle of HIV help in developing effective antiretroviral therapy?
3. In what way can an understanding of the function of chemokine receptors help in inhibiting HIV infection in the host?

3.5   Oncogenic viruses

It is estimated that 20 per cent of all human cancers have a viral aetiology (reviewed by zur Hausen, 1991), whereas the remainder are 'spontaneous' and caused by inherited or epigenetic genetic damage. Human tumour viruses comprise:

- Human papillomaviruses (HPV). These cause benign tumours of cutaneous and mucosal epithelia and are associated with skin cancers, cancer of the cervix and other anogenital cancer.
- Epstein–Barr virus (EBV). This virus causes infectious mononucleosis (glandular fever), but is also associated with several malignancies, including Burkitt's lymphoma, nasopharyngeal carcinoma and Hodgkin's disease.
- Hepatitis B and C viruses. These are associated with cirrhosis of the liver and hepatocellular carcinoma.
- Human T-lymphotrophic viruses I and II (HTLV-I and HTLV-II). These are retroviruses that cause leukaemias of T lymphocytes.

In each of these cases, the growth-transforming properties the virus has on its host cell can be attributed to one or more transforming genes. These are best characterized in the papillomaviruses. Interest in tumour viruses from an immunological perspective is twofold. First is the means by which these viruses evade the immune system, and secondly is the development of vaccines. The development of vaccines against spontaneous tumours is a formidable challenge, in part because tumour-specific target antigens must first be identified before a vaccine can be designed. Despite some successes in the area, notably in melanoma, each vaccine has to be tailor-made to suit each patient. However, tumours with a viral aetiology allow targeting of the immune response to the virus and thereby circumventing the hitherto intractable problem of identifying tumour-specific antigens.

3.5.1   *Epstein–Barr virus (EBV)*

EBV is a γ-herpesvirus with a tropism for B lymphocytes and epithelial cells of the oropharynx. This virus is famed for its growth-transforming properties of B cells. *In vitro* EBV-infected B cells become immortalized B cell lines (B-lymphoblastoid cell lines or B-LCL), and *in vivo* EBV contributes to the development of several B-cell malignances (see below). Yet 80–95 per cent of adults have EBV infection, which is life long and asymptomatic (latent). Like other herpesvirus infections, latency is interrupted by occasional recurrent episodes of viral replication. In the case of EBV, replication occurs mainly in the oropharynx allowing virions to be shed into the saliva. Primary infection of humans usually occurs during the first decade of life in which oropharyngeal epithelial cells become infected with virus transmitted from the saliva of a carrier. Circulating B lymphocytes then become infected as they traffic through the infected oropharyngeal tissue, causing the B lymphocytes to proliferate and produce new virus. EBV gains entry to B cells by the binding of its envelope glycoprotein (gp340) to CD21 on the surface of B cells, which is part of the antigen–receptor complex. Primary infections in children are usually asymptomatic, although primary infections that are delayed until adolescence can lead to infectious mononucleosis, so named after the characteristic overproduction of mononuclear cells (B cells and specific T_C cells) that appear in the blood after infection.

Infection is controlled by cytotoxic T lymphocytes that kill EBV-infected cells (Rickinson and Moss, 1997). However, a fraction of infected B cells escape, and EBV switches from the replicative (or lytic) phase of infection to the latent (non-replicative) phase in which a completely different set of genes is expressed. Latently infected B lymphocytes escape the attentions of T_C cells (section 3.2.2), thereby causing the life-long carrier state. Latently infected B cells also act as the reservoir of virus able to reinfect the oropharyngeal epithelium and lead to replication and shedding of virions into the saliva. EBV-transformed B-lymphoblastoid cell lines (B-LCL) only express latent genes and much of what we know about the immunology of EBV has come from the study of responses to (latent) viral antigens expressed by B-LCL.

Antibody responses to EBV

The host immune system plays a major role in controlling both primary infection and the carrier state. Little is known about the importance of antibody responses to EBV. Monoclonal antibodies against the major envelope protein (gp340) have been produced that are able to neutralize infectivity. If neutralizing antibodies are produced during the primary infection, they may be important in preventing subsequent infection from another carrier, although their role in controlling established infection is questionable.

Cytotoxic T-lymphocyte responses to EBV

In contrast, T_C cells play a vital role in the control of established infection – indeed, EBV is ranked alongside influenza virus as one of the best model systems in which to study T_C-cell responses in humans. It is relatively simple to obtain EBV-specific T_C cells from peripheral blood. Peripheral blood mononuclear cells (PBMC), which contain the blood lymphocytes, are cultured *in vitro* with autologous EBV-transformed B-lymphoblastoid cells (autologous = from the same donor) and IL-2. The EBV-infected B cells stimulate the proliferation of clones of memory T_C cells that have receptors specific for EBV latent antigens. The importance of these T_C cells in the control of infection is vividly illustrated by the procedure used to generate immortalized B cells from human blood cells in the laboratory. It is usually only possible to immortalize the B cells *in vitro* after the T-cell population has been selectively killed using cyclosporin, because the EBV-specific T_C cells kill any infected B cells. The relative ease with which B-LCL can be produced in the laboratory and the ease with which EBV-specific T_C cells can be obtained have allowed a detailed understanding of T_C-cell responses to latent infection. Relatively little is known about any T_C-cell responses during the replicative stage of infection of the pharyngeal epithelial cells.

Latently infected B cells express eight proteins. These include the Epstein–Barr nuclear antigens (EBNA1, -2, -3A, -3B, -3C, -LP) and the latent membrane proteins (LMP1 and LMP2). By stimulating memory T_C cells as described above, populations of T_C cells can be screened to establish which of these antigens they recognize. To do this, autologous fibroblasts are made to express individual EBV latent genes by introducing the gene into the cell (transfection) or by infecting the fibroblasts with a recombinant virus (such as vaccinia) into which EBV have been engineered. The fibroblasts are then presented to the T_C cells as 'target' cells for lysis. Killing is determined in a standard cytotoxicity assay in which release of radioactivity is measured from targets loaded intracellularly with ^{51}Cr. Using this approach it is seen that the main target antigens are EBNA3A, -3B and -3C. A smaller number of people also have T_C cells that recognize LMP2. The relative scarcity of responses to the EBNA1 antigen is thought to be due to an escape strategy used by the virus. EBNA1 has a repeated glycine–alanine motif that appears to protect the protein from antigen processing and presentation by class I MHC molecules (see section 3.2.2).

The actual epitopes recognized within these antigens can be mapped precisely by synthetic peptides corresponding to short amino acid sequences of the EBV latent antigens. So far, about 50 different epitopes have been mapped in the eight latent proteins. Over 60 per cent of these are localized in the EBNA3A, -3B and -3C antigens. A variety of class I HLA alleles have been identified as presenters (or 'restriction elements') of these epitopes. Among Caucasians, the most frequently observed restriction elements are HLA-A11, HLA-B7 and HLA-B8. As we saw in section 3.2.1, selective pressure imposed by A11-restricted T_C cells has allowed a strain harbouring a mutation in an A11 epitope to emerge. EBV also displays several means for subverting the immune system and which contribute to the maintenance of latency. These include production of a homologue of human IL-10 which serves to down-regulate T_H1 and the antiviral effects they promote, while also stimulating the proliferation of B cells (see section 3.2.3).

Control of EBV-induced malignancies

EBV infection is associated with the development of several malignancies:

- Burkitt's lymphoma (BL): a childhood malignancy of B lymphocytes that is found in equatorial Africa.
- Hodgkin's disease (HD): a malignancy of antigen-presenting cells.
- Immunoblastic lymphoma: a malignancy of B lymphocytes that occurs in immunosuppressed individuals and has re-emerged in the wake of the HIV epidemic.
- Nasopharyngeal carcinoma (NPC).

Although EBV has the ability to immortalize B lymphocytes, B-cell malignancies are extremely rare disorders in EBV-infected individuals. T_C-cell responses play the major role in surveillance, thereby preventing the emergence of malignancies. Malignancies may arise, however, if chronic immunosuppression occurs, in which case the surveillance by T_C cells is compromised. In this context, it has been noticed that the geographical distribution of Burkitt's lymphoma coincides almost exactly with the distribution of malaria. Chronic immunosuppression by *Plasmodium* infection (see section 4.4.4) may therefore predispose individuals with EBV infections to the development of lymphoma. Alternatively, latently infected cells may sustain, in addition to EBV infection, genetic damage leading to loss of recognition by T_C cells. BL cells are refractory to killing by T_C cells, which is due in part to the loss of expression by BL of surface adhesion molecules. These include ICAM-1 (intercellular

Table 3.6 Proteins of tumour viruses that interact with tumour suppressor gene products, p53 and retinoblastoma protein (Rb)

Virus	p53	Rb
EBV	EBNA-LP, LMP1	
HPV	E6	E7
Ad2, 5	E1B	E1A
HBV	HBx	
SV40	Large T	Large T

adhesion molecule-1) and LFA-3 (leucocyte function associated antigen-3), which are vital in mediating the attachment of T_C cells via LFA-1 and CD2, respectively. There is also some evidence that the class I MHC processing pathway may also be disfunctional in BL because they express less than 25 per cent of the normal levels of surface class I HLA molecules. This appears to be due to low levels of TAP expression, although how this is achieved and whether EBV is actively involved in this down-regulation remains to be elucidated. One possibility is that BL arises from B-cell progenitor cells in which the expression of HLA and adhesion molecules is normally low.

In nasopharyngeal carcinoma and Hodgkin's disease, there is a marked reduction in the expression of the latent EBV antigens EBNA3A, -3B and -3C which, as we saw earlier in this section, represent the major targets for T_C-cell recognition of EBV-infected B cells. EBNA1 is constitutively expressed in NPC and HD, although this protein possesses a long stretch of Gly–Ala repeats which has been shown to protect it from the class I MHC antigen-processing pathway (Figure 3.3). In contrast, the T_C-cell response in patients with NPC and HD is skewed towards the recognition of the LMP2 antigen, and to a lesser extent the LMP1. It has been speculated that the responses to these antigens are inherently weak and ineffective at eliminating these tumours.

The genes responsible for the growth-transforming properties of EBV are thought to reside with the EBNA-LP and LMP1 proteins, which have been shown to interact with a cellular protein, p53. This adds to a growing list of proteins produced by DNA tumour viruses that interact with p53 (see Table 3.6, and Neil *et al.*, 1997). The normal role of p53 is to arrest cells in G1 of the cell cycle after genetic damage has been sustained. However, loss of p53 function results in the cell being less able to control proliferation. Mutations in the p53 gene are the most common genetic defect in spontaneous tumours.

Table 3.7 Examples of lesions caused by human papilloma viruses

Type of lesion	Common HPV type	Anatomical location
Common wart	HPV1	Hands
Plantar wart (verruca)	HPV1	Sole of feet, toes
Plane wart	HPV3, 10	Face, arms
Mosaic warts	HPV2	Soles and heels of feet; palms, knuckles, fingers
Butchers' wart	HPV7	Hands of butchers
Anogenital warts	HPV6, 11	Genital and anal mucosa
Low-grade CIN*	HPV6, 11	Cervix
Laryngeal papillomas	HPV6, 11	Larynx
High-grade CIN	HPV16, 18	Cervix

* CIN, cervical intraepithelial neoplasia.

3.5.2 *Human papillomavirus (HPV)*

Papillomaviruses (PVs) are a family of non-enveloped, small (approximately 7.9 kbp), double-stranded DNA viruses that infect many mammals, including humans, deer, dogs, cattle and rabbits. PVs infect squamous (multilayered) mucosal and cutaneous epithelium to cause benign and self-limiting hyperproliferative lesions. In humans the host cell is the skin keratinocyte and infection leads to the formation of warts, papillomas or condylomas according to HPV type and anatomical location of infection (Table 3.7). Over 70 genetically distinct types of HPV have been discovered, each with a specific trophism for a particular type of epithelium. Interest in HPVs has stemmed from the finding that several so-called 'high risk' HPV genotypes are associated with lesions with a propensity for malignant transformation. Of major interest are HPV16 and HPV18, whose DNA can be detected in over 90 per cent of carcinomas of the cervix and other anogenital cancers. These HPV types initally cause a premalignant disease called genital intraepithelial neoplasia, of which a fraction progress to maligancy. Annually in the UK, there are approximately 4000 new cases of cervical cancer and 2000 deaths. Globally, these figures can be multiplied 100-fold, with carcinoma of the cervix being the leading cancer-associated killer of women in developing countries.

Classification of HPVs is currently based on genetic homology rather than by antigenic differences detected by antibodies (serotyping). This is because, until recently, major difficulties have been encountered in developing virus neutralization assays (discussed below). An HPV genotype is defined as having a genome that has 90 per cent or less sequence identity with other genotypes.

Owing to its serious health risk much of the research has been focused on HPV16, and to a lesser extent HPV6 (associated with low risk genital intraepithelial neoplasias and benign genital warts) and HPV1 (associated with skin warts). However, progress has been hampered by the relative paucity of HPV virions from genital lesions, particularly of the cervix. This is because assembly of the virus occurs in the most superficial layers of the epithelium which are then shed by constant exfoliation. It is also particularly difficult to propagate HPV *in vitro*. This is because HPV replication and assembly is tightly coordinated to the differentiation status of the host epithelial cell as it migrates from the basal layer toward the surface of the squamous epithelium. This differentiation process is particularly difficult to reproduce *in vitro*. For this reason, animal PVs (notably the bovine PV, cottontail rabbit PV and canine oral PV) have proved vital models in understanding the replicative cycle, growth-transforming properties and immunology of PV infection.

Much of the molecular biology of HPV has been gleaned from the BPV1 model. This is in part because relatively large quantities of virus can be obtained from bovine wart tissue, and also because BPV can infect mouse fibroblasts *in vitro*. Although infected fibroblasts cannot support full viral replication, BPV genes are transcribed and the cells do exhibit transformed growth characteristics, such as loss of anchorage to a substratum, uncontrolled proliferation, and a reduced dependency for growth factors in the tissue culture medium. All animal PVs have a broadly similar organization of genes. The genome encodes eight or nine open reading frames. These are classified into early (E1, E2, E4, E5, E6, E7 and E8) and late (L1 and L2) regions. The early regions encode polypeptides required for gene activation and cellular transformation. Those in the late region are expressed in late infection in the most superficial layers of the epithelium, and encode the only two structural proteins that make up the capsid. Owing to the small size of the genome, HPV must utilize much of the cellular enzymatic machinery to replicate itself.

The transforming properties of HPV16 have been identified as belonging to the E6 and E7 open reading frames. It should be stressed at this point that the function of these proteins is not to cause tumours as such but to release the brakes normally held on cell proliferation. By pushing the host cell into the cell cycle, HPV can create a cellular environment suitable for its own replication. In many respects the oncogenic potential of 'high risk' HPVs is an unfortunate side effect of a very effective strategy to manipulate the cell cycle. However, as with EBV, infection with HPV alone is insufficient to cause malignant progression, and several additional genetic defects caused by 'cofactors' have been implicated.

E6 and p53

There are currently two properties ascribed to E6 which contribute to cellular transformation. The first of these is binding to p53. The E6 protein shares a high degree of homology with the E6-binding proteins of two other DNA viruses that are associated with tumours in rodents. These are the E1B protein of adenovirus and the large T antigen of simian virus 40. The main function of p53 is to prevent damaged DNA from being replicated by arresting the cell in G1 of the cell cycle. Binding of E6 to p53 causes p53 to become ubiquitinylated, which targets it for cytosolic degradation by the proteasome. E6 therefore has the effect of releasing the control over cell proliferation and predisposing the cell toward a proliferative state. The blocking of p53 function also means that damaged DNA can be replicated. A second function of HPV E6 is the activation of the cellular telomerase gene. Telomerase is normally inactive in differentiated cells, but is active in self-replicating stem cells and in many immortalized cell lines. The ends of DNA molecules are unstable and need to be protected. Prokaryotes have resolved this problem by having circular genomes. Eukaryotes, on the other hand, have telomeres at their chromosomal termini which are maintained by telomerase. A telomere consists of an expendable sequence of DNA of 5–8 bp repeats. At each cell division, the telomere is progressively shortened until the telomere is lost altogether and the cell becomes senescent. The effect of telomerase activation by E6 therefore is to increase the lifespan of a proliferating cell.

E7 and retinoblastoma protein

The cellular target for the HPV E7 protein is the Rb (retinoblastoma) protein. E7 is homologous to the Rb-binding proteins of adenovirus and SV40, which are E1A and large T, respectively. The function of Rb is to block the transcription of several genes required for proliferation. This is achieved by binding to a common transcription factor, E2F. Dissociation of Rb from E2F is triggered by conformational changes brought about normally by phosphorylation of Rb, or by mutations in the *Rb* gene as seen in many spontaneous tumours. E7 binds to Rb and prevents its interaction with E2F, thereby mimicking these effects.

Immunology of HPV

It is generally accepted that HPV are weakly immunogenic during natural infection. In part, this is because HPV are non-lytic viruses; virions are shed instead from infected tissues during the normal process of exfoliation. HPV infection therefore does not normally trigger inflammatory responses required to initiate immune responses. Moreover, infected cells in the underlying layers of infected epithelium normally lack costimulatory molecules, and may serve to anergize T cells rather than activate them. In addition, there is evidence that infected cells in premalignant lesions have a reduced expression of class I MHC molecules which may allow the virus to 'hide' from T_C cells. No viral gene products respons-ible for this effect have yet been identified. When HPV-associated lesions progress to malignancy, surface class I molecules are usually absent, as is the case with many other carcinomas. However, a role for the virus in this is equivo-cal, and it is more likely that tumour cells have acquired additional mutations that modulate class I expression in-dependently of the virus. Finally, despite much effort, dir-ect evidence for HPV-specific memory T cells (both T_C cells and T_H cells) in HPV-infected donors is sparse (Nimako *et al.*, 1997), and the viral antigens that these T cells recognize are not well characterized. None the less, there is evidence that cell-mediated immunity *is* important in controlling infec-tion. This comes mainly from two lines of indirect evidence:

- Spontaneously regressing warts are actively infiltrated by leucocytes, including CD4+ and CD8+ T lymphocytes, suggesting an inflammatory reaction occurs.
- Immunosuppression (caused by immunosuppressive drugs after organ transplantation, during pregnancy, or immunodeficiencies caused by disease such as AIDS) is often associated with the emergence of skin and genital warts.

A breakthrough in understanding antibody responses has come from the discovery that the L1 major capsid protein will self-assemble into 'empty capsids' called virus-like par-ticles (VLPs) when expressed in eukaryotic cells (Lowy, 1994). The presence of the L2 minor capsid protein seems unnecessary for VLP assembly. Comparisons of VLPs with native virions show that VLPs are authentic conformational mimics. VLPs have had a major impact in two areas of HPV immunology. First, they can be used as a detection antigen for quantifying anticapsid antibody levels in patients. This has enabled sero-epidemiological studies to be performed to determine whether such antibody levels correlate with disease evolution. Secondly, VLPs of animal PVs (notably of the cottontail rabbit PV and the canine oral PV) have been used to immunize and elicit virus-neutralizing antibodies. These VLP-based vaccines have proved to be very effective, and provide 100 per cent protection to subsequent challenge from infectious viruses.

Summary of section 3.5

- EBV is a γ-herpesvirus that causes latent infections of B lymphocytes. Latency is interrupted by periodic replication and shedding from the oropharyngeal epithelial cells. T_C cells play a major role in controlling infection and the majority of carriers are asymptomatic. EBV is a model system for studying T_C-cell responses in humans; these are relatively easy to obtain and the virus can be used to immortalize B cells *in vitro*. EBV is also implicated in several malignancies, although the growth-transforming gene(s) of the virus is thought to include EBNA-LP and LMP-1 which bind to p53.

- HPVs are a family of 70 or more different genotypes that infect keratinocytes in the mucosal and cutaneous epithelium. Most lesions caused by HPVs are benign tumours (warts, condylomata, papillomas), although certain 'high risk' genotypes are associated with lesions with a risk of malignant transformation. HPV16 and HPV18, which are sexually transmitted HPVs with a tropism for anogenital mucosa, are associated with more than 95 per cent of cervical carcinomas. The transforming activities of high risk HPVs localize to the viral E6 and E7 gene products, which counteract the proliferation-limiting cellular proteins, p53 and retinoblastoma protein, respectively. No immune evasion strategies have yet been found; these are non-lytic viruses and persist largely by failing to cause inflammation.

Study problems for section 3.5

1. What are the functions of p53 and the retinoblastoma protein? What examples are there of tumour viruses that interfere with their function?

2. What are the features of EBV infection that are typical of herpesviruses and what strategies does this virus use to thwart the immune system?

Selected reading

Books for background reading

Jawetz, E., Melnick, J.L., Adelberg, E.A. and Brooks, G.F., 1995, *Reviews in Medical Microbiology*, 20th edn, London: Prentice-Hall

Krug, R.M., 1989, *The Influenza Viruses*, New York: Plenum Press

White, D. and Fenner, F., 1995, *Medical Virology,* 4th edn, San Diego: Academic Press

Zuckermann, A.J., Banatvala, J.E. and Pattison, J.R. (eds), 1996, *Principles and Practise of Clinical Virology*, 3rd edn, Chichester: John Wiley

Literature cited

Alcami, A. and Smith, G.L., 1995, Cytokine receptors encoded by poxviruses: a lesson in cytokine biology, *Immunol. Today*, **16**, 474–478

Beck, S. and Barrell, B.G., 1988, Human cytomegalovirus encodes a glycoprotein homologous to MHC class-I antigens, *Nature*, **331**, 269–272

Burgert, H.-G., 1996, Subversion of the MHC class I antigen-presentation pathway by adenoviruses and herpes simplex viruses, *Trends Microbiol.*, **4**, 107–112

Burton, D.R., 1997, A vaccine for HIV-1: the antibody perspective, *Proc. Natl. Acad. Sci. USA*, **94**, 10 018–10 023

Coffin, J.M., 1995, HIV population-dynamics *in-vivo* – implications for genetic variation, pathogenesis, and therapy, *Science*, **267**, 483–489

Cuff, S. and Ruby, J., 1996, Evasion of apoptosis by DNA viruses, *Immunol. Cell Biol.*, **74**, 527–537

Davis-Poynter, N.J. and Farrell, H.E., 1996, Masters of deception – a review of herpesvirus immune evasion strategies, *Immunol. Cell Biol.*, **74**, 513–522

de Campos-Lima, P. O., Gavioli, R., Zhang, Q.J., Wallace, L.E., Dolcetti, R., Rowe, M., Rickinson, A.B. and Masucci, M.G., 1993, HLA-A11 epitope loss isolates of Epstein–Barr virus from a highly A11+ population, *Science*, **260**, 98–100

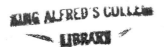

Gilbert, M.J., Riddell, S.R., Plachter, B. and Greenberg, P.D., 1996, Cytomegalovirus selectively blocks antigen processing and presentation of its intermediate-early gene product, *Nature*, **383**, 720–722

Gillet, G. and Brun, G., 1996, Viral inhibition of apoptosis, *Trends Microbiol.*, **4**, 312–317

Gooding, L.R., 1992, Virus proteins that counteract host immune defences, *Cell*, **71**, 5–7

Greene, W.C., 1991, The molecular biology of human immunodeficiency virus type 1 infection, *New Engl. J. Med.*, **324**, 308–317

Hayder, H. and Müllbacher, A., 1996, Molecular basis of immune evasion strategies by adenoviruses, *Immunol. Cell Biol.*, **74**, 505–512

Hengel, H. and Koszinowski, U.H., 1997, Interference with antigen processing by viruses, *Curr. Opin. Immunol.*, **9**, 470–476

Hill, A., Jugovic, P., York, I., Russ, G., Bennink, J., Yewdell, J., Ploegh, H. and Johnson, D., 1995, Herpes simplex virus turns off the TAP to evade host immunity, *Nature*, **375**, 411–418

Hill, A.B., 1996, Mechanisms of interference with the MHC class I-restricted pathway of antigen presentation by herpesviruses, *Immunol. Cell Biol.*, **74**, 523–526

Ho, D.D., Neumann, A.U., Perelson, A.S., Chen, W., Leonard, J.M. and Markowitz, M., 1995, Rapid turnover of plasma virions and CD4 lymphocytes in HIV-1 infection, *Nature*, **373**, 123–126

Jacobs, B.L. and Langland, J.O., 1996, When two strands are better than one – the mediators and modulators of the cellular-responses to double-stranded RNA, *Virology*, **219**, 339–349

Koup, R.A., 1994, Virus escape from CTL recognition, *J. Exp. Med.*, **180**, 779–782

Lachmann, P.J. and Davies, A., 1997, Complement and immunity to viruses, *Immunol. Rev.*, **159**, 69–77

Landolfo, S., Gribaudo, G., Angeritti, A. and Gariglio, M., 1995, Mechanisms of viral inhibition by interferons, *Pharmac. Ther.*, **65**, 415–442

Levitskaya, J., Coram, M., Levitsky, V., Imreh, S., Steigerwald-Mullen, P.M., Klein, G., Kurilla, M.G. and Masucci, M.G., 1995, Inhibition of antigen processing by the internal repeat region of the Epstein–Barr virus nuclear antigen-1, *Nature*, **375**, 685–688

Lowy, D.R., 1994, Genital human papillomavirus infection, *Proc. Natl. Acad. Sci. USA*, **91**, 2436–2440

McMichael, A., 1993, Natural selection at work on the surface of virus-infected cells, *Science*, **260**, 177

McMichael, A., 1997, How viruses hide from T cells, *Trends Microbiol.*, **5**, 211–212

Mellors, J.W., Rinaldo, C.R., Gupta, P., White, R.M., Todd, J.A. and Kingsley, L.A., 1996, Prognosis in HIV-1 infection predicted by the quantity of virus in plasma, *Science*, **272**, 1167–1170

Moore, K.W., Vieira, P., Fiorentino, D.F., Trounstine, M.L., Khan, T.A. and Mossman, T.R., 1990, Homology of cytokine synthesis inhibitory factor (IL-10) to the Epstein-Barr virus gene BCRF-1, *Science*, **248**, 1230–1234

Neil, J.C., Cameron, E.R. and Baxter, E.W., 1997, p53 and tumour viruses: catching the guardian off-guard, *Trends Microbiol.*, **5**, 115–120

Nimako, M., Fiander, A.N., Wilkinson, G.W.G., Borysiewicz, L.K. and Man, S., 1997, Human papillomavirus-specific cytotoxic T lymphocytes in patients with cervical intra-epithelial neoplasia grade III, *Cancer Res.*, **57**, 4855–4861

Parker, C.E. and Gould, K.G., 1996, Influenza A virus – a model for viral antigen presentation to cytotoxic T lymphocytes, *Sem. Virol.*, **7**, 61–73

Perelson, A.S., Essunger, P., Cao, Y., Vesanen, M., Hurley, A., Saksela, K., Markowitz, M. and Ho, D.D., 1997, Decay characteristics of HIV-1-infected compartments during combination therapy, *Nature*, **387**, 188–191

Rickinson, A.B. and Moss, D.J., 1997, Human cytotoxic T lymphocyte responses to Epstein–Barr virus infection, *Annu. Rev. Immunol.*, **15**, 405–431

Rotem-Yehudar, R., Groettrud, M., Soza, A., Kluetzel, P.M., Ehrlich, R., 1996, LMP-associated proteolytic activities and TAP-dependent peptide transport for class I MHC molecules are suppressed in cell lines transformed by the highly oncogenic adenovirus 12, *J. Exp. Med.*, **183**, 499–514

Schuurman, R., Nijhuis, M., Vanleeuwen, R., Schipper, P., Dejong, D., Collis, P., Danner, S.A., Mulder, J. Loveday, C., Christopherson, C., Kwok, S., Sninsky, J. and Boucher, C.A.B., 1995, Rapid changes in human-immunodeficiency-virus type-1 RNA load and appearance of drug-resistant virus populations in persons treated with lamivudine (3TC), *J. Infect. Dis.*, **171**, 1411–1419

Smith, G.L., 1996, Virus proteins that bind cytokines, chemokines or interferons, *Curr. Opin. Immunol.*, **8**, 467–471

Spriggs, M.K., 1994, Cytokine and cytokine receptor genes 'captured' by viruses, *Curr. Opin. Immunol.*, **6,** 526–529

Townsend, A.R.M. and Bodmer, H., 1989, Antigen recognition by class I restricted T cells, *Annu. Rev. Immunol.*, **7,** 601–624

Tyring, S.K., 1995, Interferons: biochemistry and mechanisms of action, *Am. J. Obstet. Gynecol.*, **172**, 1350–1353

Wei, X.P., Ghosh, S.K., Taylor, M.E., Johnson, V.A., Emini, E.A., Deutsch, P., Lifson, J.D., Bonhoeffer, S., Nowak, M.A., Hahn, B.H., Saag, M.S. and Shaw, G.M., 1995, Viral dynamics in human-immunodeficiency-virus type-1 infection, *Nature*, **373**, 117–122

Wiertz, E.J.H.J., Tortorella, D., Bogyo, M., Yu, J., Mothes, W., Jones, T.R., Rapoport, T.A. and Ploegh, H.L., 1996, Sec61-mediated transfer of a membrane protein from the endoplasmic reticulum to the proteasome for destruction, *Nature*, **384**, 432–438

Wiley, D.C., Wilson, I.A. and Skehel, J.J., 1981, Structural identification of the antibody-binding sites of Hong Kong influenza haemagglutinin and their involvement in antigenic variation, *Nature*, **289**, 373–378

zur Hausen, H., 1991, Viruses in human cancers, *Science*, **254**, 1167

4 Parasitic Infections

4.1 Introduction

Strictly speaking the term 'parasite' can be applied to any organism that is capable of infecting a host but, by convention, is usually restricted to eukaryotic protozoa and helminth worms and this chapter will consider only these groups. Until relatively recently the immunology of parasitic infections was regarded as something separate from the immunology of viral and bacterial infections and parasites have usually been omitted from textbooks of microbiology. However, things are changing and more recent texts are less restrictive about what constitutes a microorganism than the older ones. The most useful categorization of infectious agents is to regard them as either microparasites or macroparasites. Microparasites are small, have short generation times and multiply within their vertebrate hosts, whereas macroparasites tend to be large and do not multiply within their vertebrate hosts. Microparasites include viruses, bacteria and protozoa which, because they are capable of multiplying indefinitely in their hosts, usually at a logarithmic rate, present an immediate threat that must be countered by a rapid and effective immune response. Infections with microparasites, therefore, tend to be acute but of short duration and characterized by an effective immune response that brings the existing infection under control and may also prevent reinfection. Infections with macroparasites are largely dependent on the number of infectious stages ingested or injected as one infectious stage gives rise to only one adult worm. Infections tend to build up slowly and, unless the worm burden is very large, usually cause little harm and are seldom immediately life-threatening. The immune response only comes into play at a relatively late stage of the infection and tends to prevent reinfection of the already infected host rather than curtailing the ongoing infection, a phenomenon known as concomitant immunity. Infections with macroparasites are typically of long duration and accompanied by a slowly developing immune response which may only be effective while the host is infected. Immunity quickly fades and does not usually protect against subsequent challenge. However, like all generalizations, there are so many exceptions to these principles that each

Table 4.1 Parasites discussed in this chapter, the diseases caused and their prevalence (WHO figures)

Genus	Species	Disease	Prevalence (thousands)
Leishmania	*tropica, major, mexicana braziliensis, donovani, chagasi*	Leishmaniasis	12 000
Trypanosoma	*cruzi*	Chagas' disease	18 000
Trypanosoma	*gambiense, rhodesiense*	Sleeping sickness	300
Plasmodium	*falciparum, vivax, malariae, ovale*	Malaria	350 000
Schistosoma	*mansoni, japonicum haematobium*	Schistosomiasis	200 000
Wuchereria Brugia	*bancrofti, malayi*	Lymphatic filariasis	120 000
Onchocerca	*volvulus*	Onchocerciasis	18 000

individual infection must be considered separately. The important message here is that, as far as the immunology is concerned, protozoan infections resemble bacterial and viral infections more closely than they resemble helminth infections. The grouping of protozoa and helminths together is therefore largely artificial but is maintained here for traditional reasons and as a matter of convenience.

Humans are remarkably susceptible to infections with parasites and harbour over 30 species of protozoa and over 60 species of helminths but, fortunately, only a few of these are common and even fewer normally cause serious disease. However, in recent years there have been increasing numbers of reports of new and hitherto relatively harmless parasitic infections that have become life-threatening in individuals infected with HIV or undergoing immunosuppressive therapy. It is beyond the scope of this chapter to discuss all the important parasitic infections and coverage will be restricted to what are known as the 'six diseases' identified by the World Health Organization in the 1970s as the most important infections in its Tropical Diseases Research Programme. Of these, leishmaniasis, African and South American trypanosomiasis, malaria, schistosomiasis and filariasis are caused by parasites, the sixth being leprosy. Table 4.1 lists the parasites covered in this chapter, diseases caused and prevalence. These parasitic diseases are the ones that have received most attention and about which most is known, but this does not mean that other parasites do not present serious problems or that parasites are not important outside the tropics and the reader is referred to standard textbooks of parasitology and tropical medicine listed in the bibliography for further information. In addition to their effects on humans, parasites present a continual threat to domesticated animals all over the world and the losses caused in terms of loss of productivity and premature mortality run into many millions of pounds every year.

4.2   Structure and classification

4.2.1   *Structure and classification of parasitic protozoa*

Protozoa are by definition single-celled eukaryotic organisms. This means that they consist of single cells containing all the components found in any eukaryotic cell. Some forms have sexual stages, permitting a degree of genetic recombination, but in all cases actual multiplication occurs at a well-defined doubling rate, usually by binary fission, thus a single parasite can quickly give rise to large numbers of daughter cells. Many of the parasitic species have complex life cycles involving several different stages, which often differ biochemically and antigenically from one another. From an immunological viewpoint, the most important structure of any parasitic protozoan is its cell membrane, which acts as the interface between parasite and host. These membranes are frequently embedded or covered with a variety of molecules, some of which are possible targets for immunological attack and some of which are involved in immune evasion.

The classification of the parasitic protozoa is currently in a state of flux, mainly because of difficulties in establishing the affinities of the free-living relatives of parasitic forms (see Cox, 1998). Organisms that have been traditionally regarded as protozoa (i.e. unicellular eukaryotic organisms) are now being divided between several kingdoms, but only one, the kingdom Protozoa, contains the parasites discussed in this chapter. The classification given in Table 4.2 is a traditional one that can be regarded as a working compromise and is compatible with classifications given in textbooks and used in abstracting journals.

4.2.2   *Structure and classification of parasitic helminths*

There are three important groups of helminth worms: nematoda or roundworms, flukes or flatworms, and cestoda or

Table 4.2   An outline classification of the parasitic protozoa of humans considered in this chapter

Empire	Eukaryota
Kingdom	Protozoa Unicellular, plasmodial or colonial colourless phagotrophic organisms that typically possess tubular cristate mitochondria, Golgi bodies and peroxisomes
Phylum	Euglenozoa Unicellular flagellates with 1–4 flagella, Golgi body and mitochondria
Class	Kinetoplastidea Unicellular flagellates with 1–2 flagella, and prominent kinetoplast (DNA-containing body) within a single mitochondrion
Order	Trypanosomatida Genera *Leishmania*, *Trypanosoma*
Phylum	Sporozoa (Apicomplexa) Unicellular organisms possessing at some stage an apical complex composed of polar rings, rhoptries, micronemes and typically a conoid; elaborate life cycles involving a sexual process; all parasites
Class	Haematozoa Sexual stages in blood of vertebrate host and in blood-sucking arthropod
Order	Haemosporida Genus *Plasmodium*

tapeworms. All are highly evolved metazoa with sexual reproduction and complex life cycles often involving an intermediate host. The most significant features with respect to immunity are their size, which ranges from about 10 mm to over 10 m, and the complexity of their outer surfaces which contain numerous molecules that are involved both as possible targets for immune attack and for the evasion of the immune response. The size of helminth worms means that they cannot easily be phagocytosed or attacked by antibody. Antibody-dependent cell-mediated cytotoxicity, ADCC (see section 1.5), often involving eosinophils as well as macrophages is the main mechanism whereby immunity is effected.

The classification of parasitic worms, which is based on solid zoological principles, has remained relatively stable and the classification outlined in Table 4.3 is widely accepted and used in textbooks and in abstracting journals (see Gibson, 1998).

Table 4.3 An outline classification of the parasitic helminths of humans considered in this chapter

Phylum	Platyhelminthes (flatworms)
	Bilaterally symmetrical, dorsoventrally flattened, hermaphrodite, acoelomate worms. Three parasitic classes: Monogenea (mainly parasites of fishes), Cestoidea (tapeworms) and Trematoda (flukes) of which only the last two contain parasites of humans
Class	Trematoda (flukes).
	Adults possess oral and ventral suckers; adults parasitic in vertebrates; indirect life cycle involving mollusc and possibly additionally other invertebrates
Subclass	Digenea
	Order Strigeida; genus *Schistosoma*
Phylum	Nematoda (roundworms)
	Bilaterally symmetrical, unsegmented pseudocoelomates; sexes separate
Class	Secernentea
	Possess posterior phasmid chemoreceptors
	Superfamily Filarioidea,
	Family Onchocercidae,
	Genera *Brugia, Onchocerca, Wuchereria*

4.3 Immune responses to parasites

Parasites are highly evolved and remarkably adaptable organisms, all of which have developed several ways to evade the host's immune response including the capacity to depress the activities of part of the immune system. The net result is that the host becomes a battlefield between the parasite and the immune response. The consequences of the parasites' struggle to survive in a hostile environment are that infections tend to be long and chronic, the control of the immune response becomes disrupted, the immune response becomes misdirected and damage is caused to the host instead of the parasite. In addition, the infections are accompanied by immunosuppression to superimposed antigens. This immunosuppression is brought about partly by the parasites and partly by the activities of the host as it attempts to turn off unproductive and possibly dangerous immune responses.

Immune responses to parasites are so complex and so diverse that it is only within the last decade that it has been possible to take a synoptic view of immunity and immunopathology as a whole. This is because our increasing understanding of the roles of T_H1 and T_H2 cytokines has enabled

us to dissect the immune response with great precision (see
section 1.6; and also Cox and Liew, 1992; Mosmann and
Sad, 1996; Allen and Maizels, 1997; Constant and Bottomly,
1997; Romagnani, 1997). Among the T_H1 cytokines, IL-2 controls MHC-restricted target cell killing and IFN-γ controls
the activation of macrophages. The products of activated
macrophages include reactive oxygen intermediates (ROI),
nitric oxide (NO), tumour necrosis factor (TNF) and IL-12,
the last induces the production of IFN-γ by natural killer
(NK) cells and constitutes a feedback loop. Together these
activities comprise what is known as the cell-mediated, or
antibody-independent, arm of the immune response. The
T_H2 cytokines IL-4 and IL-5 control the production of antibodies and this comprises the antibody-dependent arm of
the immune response. It is important, however, to realize
that the two arms of the immune response do not operate
in isolation but are parts of a network of cytokines working both constructively and antagonistically. For example,
IL-5 is involved in the differentiation and activation of
eosinophils, IFN-γ controls some antibody activity and IL-4
inhibits some macrophage activities. Parasites are, therefore, enmeshed in this network of immune responses and at
one time it was believed that, in protozoan infections, T_H1
cell cytokines led to protective cell-mediated immunity and
T_H2 cytokines contributed to pathology, whereas in helminth
infections the reverse was the case. This was a useful start-
ing point and one from which most of our current understanding of immunity to parasites stems. However, these
assumptions about immunity to protozoa and helminths no
longer stand up to detailed analysis and it is now known
that both T_H1 and T_H2 cytokines are involved in some aspect
of protection in the majority of parasitic infections and that
the importance of different cytokines varies from species to
species and from stage to stage of the life cycle. Nevertheless, the significance of our understanding of the cytokine
network is that in all parasitic infections it is becoming
possible to disentangle factors responsible for protection
from those responsible for pathology and to link these differences to different cytokine profiles. This knowledge is an
essential prerequisite for the development of vaccines and
ways of ameliorating adverse immune reactions.

The study of immunity to parasitic infections has not
merely followed the trends seen in other infections but has
actually led to pioneering work in a number of areas of
immunology. Various parasitic infections have been used to
test the T_H1/T_H2 paradigm, especially in humans, to establish the roles of NK cells, IL-12 and NO, to investigate the

relationships between immunity and immunopathology, and to explore the roles of alternative immune responses during infections. In this context, the role of NO in the immunology and immunopathology of parasitic infections has become paramount (see James, 1995; Clark and Rockett, 1996; MacMicking *et al.*, 1997).

As pointed out above, the life cycles of parasites are very complex and most involve a series of antigenically different stages occupying different sites in the host. In order to counteract such highly evolved and elusive targets the immune responses must be equally complex and the real problem is establishing which parts are involved in protection, counterprotection or pathology or are simply irrelevant. Immunity to parasitic infections does not involve any special or specific mechanisms but it is the sequential or concurrent occurrence of a number of immune mechanisms, some involved in protection and some involved in counterprotection, that contribute to the complexity of the immune responses seen. The mechanisms most frequently involved in protective immunity to parasites are killing by activated macrophages, antibody with or without complement, and ADCC. Cytotoxic CD8+ cells are rarely involved. However, different mechanisms may operate at different sites and at different times during the infection and protection can only be achieved by coordinated control of the different components of the immune system. This control is confounded by the fact that most parasites exert their own control on the immune system in order to manipulate the immune response in such a way as to enhance the chances of their own survival.

Another complication of parasitic infections is that, because of the nature of the complex life cycles of many parasites, the immunological mechanisms that bring the primary infection under control are not necessarily the same as those that protect the host against subsequent exposure. This is particularly marked in the cases of malaria and schistosomiasis.

Our understanding of immunity to the parasitic infections of humans (and also domesticated animals) is remarkably limited and much of what we know has been derived from laboratory *in vitro* studies and *in vivo* animal models. Such studies are, at best, merely indicative of what might actually be happening in humans and, at worst, seriously misleading. Notwithstanding the important clues that have been derived from such studies, it is important to bear in mind that in any infection of long duration caused by organisms expressing numerous antigenic epitopes there will inevitably be a plethora of immune responses and that these will inevitably be detected using standard laboratory procedures. Many of the conclusions drawn, and concepts that have been widely promulgated, have been overoptimistically interpreted and this is important to remember when reading the primary and secondary literature.

It is important to know something about parasite life cycles as well as the mechanisms of immunity but there is a tendency among some immunologists to dismiss details of the structure and complexity of life cycles as irrelevant. However, a knowledge of the nature of the parasites and their life cycles is not trivial as it is impossible to understand the mechanisms underlying protective and counterprotective immune responses unless these seemingly unimportant details are understood. This is particularly important in the application of knowledge to the development of vaccines and to ways of ameliorating pathology. For further information, the reader is referred to Warren (1993), Wakelin (1996) and Cox and Wakelin (1998).

4.4   Immunity to parasitic protozoa

As pointed out earlier, protozoa are microparasites that multiply within their vertebrate hosts at a genetically determined doubling rate and the only way that this multiplication can be halted is by the generation of an immune response. However, this does not necessarily eliminate the infection because protozoan parasites have evolved subtle ways to avoid eliciting and to evade immunological responses. As a consequence, the characteristic pattern of infection involves a latent period, a period of logarithmic increase in the number of organisms, a crisis, and a rapid or gradual decline in parasite numbers leading to a long-lasting chronic infection often with subsequent recrudescences. Typically, infections are accompanied by immunosuppression and a number of immunological changes, many of which have little to do with protection and which sometimes mirror recovery but do not necessarily reflect any protective mechanism.

Several species of parasitic protozoa inhabit macrophages at some stage during their life cycles. These include the important parasites of humans, *Leishmania* spp., *Trypanosoma cruzi* and *Toxoplasma gondii*, of which only the first two will be considered further in this chapter. *Leishmania* spp. are totally dependent on macrophages whereas *T. cruzi* is also able to infect other nucleated cell types. Each has evolved mechanisms for avoiding destruction by macrophages; leishmanias survive in the fused phagolysosome and

T. cruzi escapes from the phagosome into the macrophage cytoplasm and both possess enzymes that counteract the toxic products in the phagolysosome (reviewed by Mauel, 1996). These parasites therefore avoid destruction by macrophages, one of the main arms of the innate immune system, but cannot, however, survive in IFN-γ activated macrophages.

Some of the most important protozoan parasites inhabit the human bloodstream. These are the African trypanosomes, *Trypanosoma brucei gambiense* and *T. b. rhodesiense*, the South American trypanosome, *Trypanosoma cruzi*, and the malaria parasites, *Plasmodium falciparum*, *P. malariae*, *P. ovale* and *P. vivax*. *Babesia* spp., which are important pathogens of cattle and other domesticated animals, are rare as are accidental infections of humans and will not be considered further in this chapter. The bloodstream is a potentially hostile environment for parasites, as there they are continually exposed to components of the immune system, particularly antibodies and phagocytic cells.

4.4.1 *Immunology of leishmaniasis*

Human leishmaniasis, caused by more than 20 species of *Leishmania*, occurs in three forms, cutaneous, mucocutaneous and visceral, but these categories are not absolute. In the Old World, cutaneous leishmaniasis is caused by *L. major, L. tropica* and *L. aethiopica*, which also causes diffuse cutaneous leishmaniasis, and the visceral form by *L. donovani*. In the New World several species are involved, the most important being *L. mexicana* which causes cutaneous leishmaniasis, *L. braziliensis* which causes mucocutaneous leishmaniasis and *L. chagasi* which is the equivalent of *L. donovani*. *Leishmania* spp. are transmitted by sandflies. Infective metacyclic stages are injected into the skin when a sandfly feeds and the parasites enter macrophages where they round up and become amastigotes. These divide by binary fission until the macrophage bursts and the liberated parasites enter other macrophages; this is repeated indefinitely, causing either a local cutaneous or mucocutaneous lesion or a generalized infection if the parasites are carried to the viscera. Sandflies become infected when they feed and take up infected macrophages or free amastigotes. For further information see Ashford and Bates (1998).

There is considerable evidence for the acquisition of immunity to leishmaniasis in humans and the majority of individuals infected with the cutaneous forms eventually recover, although this may take several years. Immunity to diffuse cutaneous leishmaniasis, if it occurs at all, is even

slower to develop and, without treatment, there is little or
no immunity to the visceral forms. *Leishmania major* and
L. donovani have been extensively studied, partly because
of the ease with which they can be maintained in genetically characterized laboratory mice (reviewed by Liew and
O'Donnell, 1993). The *Leishmania major*–mouse model is
the paradigm for cutaneous leishmanial infections and comparisons with human infections suggest that the immune
responses involved are similar. *Leishmania* parasites multiply within normal macrophages but are killed by IFN-γ activated macrophages through a nitric oxide (NO)-dependent
mechanism. Tumour necrosis factor and TNF-inducers up-
regulate the IFN-γ induced NO killing. In experimental infections, NO activity is down-regulated by IL-4 and IL-10,
thus strains of mice that have high levels of IFN-γ and low
levels of IL-4 and IL-10 are resistant to infection whereas
in susceptible strains the reverse is the case. The outcome
of the immune response depends on which of the two subsets of T lymphocytes is activated, T_H1 cells producing IFN-
γ are protective while T_H2 cells producing IL-4 and IL-10
are counterprotective. IL-12 also plays a major role in immunity to leishmaniasis in mice as it initiates the production of
IFN-γ, by way of NK cells, and drives the immune response
towards the protective T_H1 pole, whereas IL-4 drives the
response towards the counterprotective T_H2 pole. Overall, it
is the actual levels of T_H1 and T_H2 cytokines that are crucial
to the outcome of the response (see Figure 4.1 and Liew and
O'Donnell, 1993; Nabors, 1997).

The pathology associated with cutaneous leishmaniasis
is largely concerned with large non-healing or slowly healing ulcers at the site of the infection. The pathology is actually enhanced by the production of cytokines that attract
macrophages to the site in what should be a normal protective inflammatory response but which, instead of destroying
the parasites, actually provides more of them to be invaded.

Differences in the roles of T_H1 and T_H2 subsets in human
leishmanial infections, although similar, are not so clear cut
as in mice (Kemp *et al.*, 1996). In patients with fulminating
L. donovani infections, IL-4 and IL-10 levels tend to be high
and IFN-γ levels low, but after treatment IFN-γ levels rise
suggesting a shift from a T_H2 to a T_H1 response. In chronic
mucocutaneous infections IL-4 levels are high and in re-
solving cutaneous infections IFN-γ levels are high. This is
in accordance with clinical observations in which the development of strong delayed-type hypersensitivity (DTH),
indicating macrophage activation, correlates with recovery
from cutaneous leishmaniasis and the absence of DTH cor-

Figure 4.1

Schematic representation of the balance of cytokines that determine the outcome of leishmaniasis infections.

The upper part of the figure shows the cytokines involved in the protective immune response which leads to the production of nitric oxide (NO) and parasite killing. The lower part shows the cytokines involved in the production of irrelevant antibody and also the counterprotective immune response in which IL-4 and IL-10 inhibit the production of NO and permit parasite survival. This figure is purely diagrammatic and does not indicate the precise points at which each cytokine functions. For further information see the text.

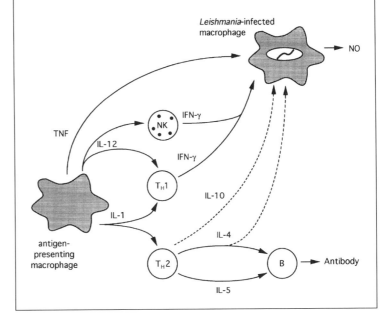

relates with diffuse cutaneous leishmaniasis. High levels of non-protective antibodies, indicating high T_H2 cell and low T_H1 cell activity, are seen in ongoing visceral leishmaniasis, again supporting the murine paradigm.

A number of experimental vaccines against leishmaniasis have been developed and there have also been some encouraging results in humans. Self-protection by exposure of inconspicuous parts of the body to the bites of sandflies has been practised for centuries and crude vaccines, using killed cultured forms, have been very promising in large field trials. In laboratory models, the development of vaccines has reached a very sophisticated level and protective antigens have been cloned and expressed in *Escherichia coli* and *Salmonella* vectors and as DNA vaccines (see Handman, 1997). However, currently there are no commercial vaccines in the pipeline, although the WHO is optimistic that eventually some will be available for clinical trials (Modabber, 1995).

4.4.2 *Immunology of African trypanosomiasis*

African trypanosomiasis affects humans in a wide belt across sub-Saharan Africa causing the disease known as sleeping sickness. Trypanosomes are flagellated protozoa belonging to the same order as the leishmanial parasites and are transmitted from host to host by tsetse flies. The species of trypanosomes that infect humans are *Trypanosoma brucei gambiense*, causing West-African or chronic sleeping sickness, and *T. b. rhodesiense*, causing East-African or acute sleeping sickness. Both are closely related to *T. b. brucei* and other trypanosomes of wildlife and domesticated animals that do not infect humans. In actual fact little is known about immunity to trypanosomes in humans and, because of the similarities between these parasites, *T. b. brucei*, which easily infects mice and other laboratory animals, has been widely used as a model for both the human and animal disease. The infection in humans begins when an infected tsetse fly bites and injects metacyclic trypanosomes into the skin. Trypanosomes multiply at the site of the bite causing the development of a chancre characterized by the infiltration of cells of various kinds. The significance of the chancre is not at all clear, but while the trypanosomes are dividing in this site they may acquire some of the features that later permit them to survive in the blood. The trypanosomes then leave the chancre as long slender forms and multiply in the blood plasma and extravascular fluids by repeated binary fission. This phase of multiplication does not proceed unabated but is periodically curtailed and the parasite levels drop only to rise again, resulting in characteristic irregular waves of parasitaemia which may continue indefinitely (Figure 4.2). Eventually some of the trypanosomes stop dividing and assume a short stumpy appearance and are taken up by a tsetse fly within which a further phase of development takes place resulting in the formation of metacyclic forms in the salivary glands of the fly and the potential to initiate a new infection. For further information see Seed (1998).

From an immunological viewpoint the waves of parasitaemia are very interesting as they represent the expression of different antigenic variants by the trypanosomes. Every bloodstream trypanosome is totally encased in a thick glycoprotein coat, the variant surface glycoprotein (VSG), of

Figure 4.2

Schematic representation of antigenic variation in an African trypanosome infection.
Trypanosomes expressing an initial variant surface glycoprotein (VSG) multiply in the blood,
the VSG is recognized by the immune system and the trypanosomes are destroyed.
However, trypanosomes expressing another VSG replace those that have been destroyed
and this pattern is repeated indefinitely. In this diagram the successive peaks of
parasitaemia A–D represent different VSGs and each peak is accompanied by the
production of antibodies to that VSG but to no other. Over the course of the infection there
is an accumulation of antibodies with different specificities each representing a response to
a particular VSG.

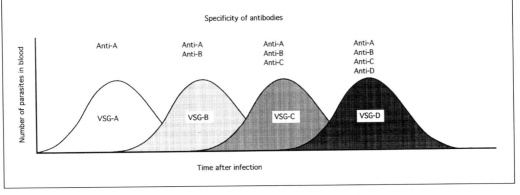

which there is an almost limitless repertoire of antigenically
different forms (Figure 4.3). The mechanism of antigenic
variation is well understood. Every trypanosome possesses
at least 1000 basic copy VSG genes which are copied and
expressed when transposed to a chromosome telomeric site.
However, only one gene is expressed at a time and, as the
majority of trypanosomes in a population in the blood at
any one time express one particular gene, the population is
defined as a variable antigen type (VAT). Individual trypanosomes can shed one and express another VSG and this
variant antigen switching occurs spontaneously about every
100 divisions. Therefore, in every population there are small
numbers of trypanosomes that possess variants that differ
from the predominant one. During the course of an infection the trypanosomes multiply in the blood and, as they
are exposed in the bloodstream and the surface coat is highly
immunogenic, they elicit a rapid and effective immune response and are destroyed by antibodies specific to the major
VSG. However, trypanosomes with different VSGs are not
affected and a population of one of these multiplies until it
in its turn is recognized and destroyed and replaced by
yet other trypanosomes with another VSG. The actual number of VATs varies between isolates and is thought to be
determined, in part at least, by the nature of the population

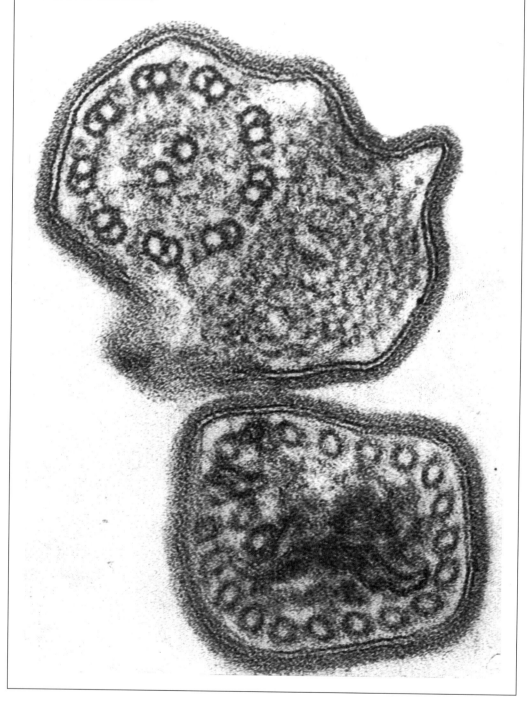

Figure 4.3

Electronmicrograph of *Trypanosoma brucei* showing the thick glycoprotein coat that consists mainly of the variant surface glycoprotein (VSG) (photograph by courtesy of Professor K. Vickerman).

injected by the tsetse fly. The surface coat consisting of the VSG is lost when taken up by a tsetse fly and regenerated in the salivary glands and there is some indication that the number and subsequent sequence of the variants passed out reflect those taken in. The nature of subsequent VATs is also possibly affected by events occurring in the chancre. The mechanisms of antigenic variation are discussed by Barry (1997).

Immunity to infection is antibody mediated and there is no evidence of any significant protective cell-mediated immunity. T-cell-independent IgM targeted to a particular VSG is the main antibody involved in human and animal infections and the actual killing mechanism involves agglutination, antibody facilitated phagocytosis with or without complement, mainly by the Kupffer cells (macrophages) of the liver, and some complement-mediated lysis. Each wave of parasitaemia is followed by a rise of IgM antibodies specific to the VSG predominant in that wave. The involvement of IgM is typical of first exposures to new antigens and to the host the generation of new VSGs effectively represents a series of antigenically distinct challenges. There is some IgG produced but its role in immunity is not fully understood.

As well as antigenic variation, trypanosomes evade the immune response and enhance their chances of survival by a generalized trypanosome-induced immunosuppression of both B-cell and T-cell function (see Mansfield, 1995; Sternberg, 1998). Immunosuppression is mediated by 'suppressor macrophages' that are characterized by enhanced activity and the production of prostaglandin-E$_2$ (PG-E$_2$), NO and ROI which, in other infections, can be protective but, in this case, are immunosuppressive. NO is capable of killing trypanosomes *in vitro* but cannot do so in the blood where haemoglobin acts as an NO sink. Several trypanosome-derived factors, including parts of the VSG molecule, activate the production of IFN-γ which actually stimulates the growth of trypanosomes. Overall, the various events that occur during a trypanosome infection represent massive disruption of the cytokine network and trypanosomes are instrumental in causing this disruption and are also caught up in its results. The pathology associated with trypanosomiasis is largely due to this disruption and to the destruction of trypanosomes, which results in the release of a number of poorly characterized internal and external antigens and toxins. These initiate immune complex-mediated damage and the production of pharmacologically active substances which affect smooth muscle contraction and vascular permeability. Trypanosome infections are also accompanied by massive polyclonal B-cell activation resulting in the production of large amounts of non-specific IgM. These phenomena have been extensively studied in experimental infections and similar processes appear to occur in humans.

Because of the phenomenon of antigenic variation, the prospects of developing a vaccine are poor at present. However, in some geographical areas there is only a limited repertoire of VATs so it is conceivable that a cocktail vaccine containing all the relevant variants might be possible. In addition, there is some evidence that a strong immunity can develop against conserved regions of the VSG and this might form a basis for a vaccine.

4.4.3   *Immunology of Chagas' disease (New World trypanosomiasis)*

Chagas' disease, caused by the trypanosome *Trypanosoma cruzi*, is confined to South and Central America where, as well as humans, it infects over 150 species of mammals. The infection is transmitted by triatome 'kissing' bugs and the infection begins when infective stages of the parasite are passed out with the bug's faeces while it is feeding and rubbed into the bite. There is a local reaction called a chagoma and parasites first multiply at the site of the bite and then circulate as trypanosomes in the blood for a short time before entering macrophages. Here they round up and become amastigotes (morphologically similar to the stages seen in *Leishmania* spp.) which survive in the macrophage by escaping from the phagolysosome and multiplying in the cytoplasm of the cell. Eventually they escape from the macrophages as trypanosomes and enter muscle cells, particularly cardiac muscle, nerve cells and other nucleated cells. Small numbers of trypanosome forms also circulate in the blood, from which they are taken up by an appropriate bug when it feeds and the cycle is completed when metacyclic forms appear in the hind gut, from which they are extruded when the bug feeds. Chagas' disease is insidious and is usually acquired by children, most of whom experience little more than a localized swelling and a transient fever. In about 2–8 per cent of those afflicted the infection may at this stage be acute and life threatening. However, in the majority of cases the infection is chronic and life long, suggesting the acquisition of immunity but a failure to control the infection completely. For further information see Miles (1998).

Much of what we know about immunity to *T. cruzi* has come from experiments with mice, in which the outcome is influenced by the genetic makeup of both the parasite and host, and a number of immunological defence mechanisms have been identified. Unlike the African trypanosomes, *T. cruzi* does not possess a thick external coat nor does it undergo antigenic variation and there is actually little genetic variability.

There are two possible targets for immune attack, the intracellular amastigote form in the macrophage and the trypanosome in the blood. Most is known about what happens to the intracellular parasites. From *in vivo* and *in vitro* studies it is clear that activated macrophages and the production of NO constitute the major defence mechanism. However, a variety of immune evasion mechanisms operate during *T. cruzi* infections and these contribute both to the longevity of the infection and to the pathological changes associated with it. As well as evading macrophage destruction by escaping from the phagolysosome and occupying non-phagocytic cells, the parasites themselves produce a number of molecules that interfere with various components of the immune system, including lymphocyte receptors, and also induce the production of IL-10 and transforming growth factor-β (TGF-β) that inhibit macrophage activity. There is also a generalized parasite-induced immunosuppression which is most obvious during the acute phase but is also evident during the chronic phase of the infection. Immunosuppression involves many components of the immune system including the depression of cytokine production and is associated with the effector phase of the immune response, particularly IFN-γ activation of macrophages.

Immunity to the bloodstream trypanosomes involves antibody, initially IgM and later IgG, but the actual mechanism of parasite killing, especially the role of complement, is controversial. Trypanosomes are resistant to complement lysis and this presumably helps the parasite to evade the immune response. *T. cruzi* also expresses molecules that mimic those of host cells, thus inhibiting immune recognition, but unfortunately, the inevitable outcome of the possession of shared antigens is to elicit autoimmunity which is characteristic of this infection.

Chronic infections are accompanied by a gradual destruction of infected muscle and nerve cells which may result in cardiac failure and loss of control of the digestive system 20–30 or more years later. During this time, the infection may be reactivated to its acute form by immunosuppressive therapy or concomitant infections. This indicates an unstable immunity operating at the limits of its efficacy. In the later stages of Chagas' disease the heart is often infiltrated by lymphocytes. The mechanisms of pathogenesis are not

fully understood. The destruction of host cells is an autoimmune phenomenon, but whether it is initiated by antigens
of host or parasite origin or both is not at all clear. Some
parasite antigens are adsorbed on to host cells which are
then destroyed by the immune response releasing further
antigens and accelerating the autoimmune reactions. There
are also antigens shared by the parasite and host neural and
cardiac cells, for example laminin and myosin are found in
both the heart and the trypanosome surface, and there are
also cross-reacting ribosomal proteins (see DosReis, 1997;
Reed, 1998).

In summary, immunity to *T. cruzi* involves some of the
most complex immunological responses encountered in any
infection and the nature of the interplay between immunity,
immune evasion and autoimmunity is likely to take many
years to elucidate. In the meantime, although some experimental vaccines have been developed, the possibility of a
protective vaccine that does not cause any autoimmunity
against this important human pathogen seems remote.

4.4.4　*Immunology of malaria*

Malaria is one of the most important diseases in the world
in terms of mortality and morbidity. Humans harbour four
species of malaria parasite, *Plasmodium falciparum*, *P. vivax*,
P. malariae and *P. ovale*, of which *P. falciparum* which
causes malignant tertian malaria is the most dangerous. The
life cycle of the malaria parasites is complex (Figure 4.4).
P. falciparum infections begin when the infective stages,
sporozoites, are injected by a mosquito directly into a cap-
illary in the skin. The sporozoites circulate in the blood
for 30–45 min before actively entering liver hepatocytes
where repeated nuclear divisions occur, a process called
exoerythrocytic schizogony, resulting in the production of
about 30 000 uninucleate merozoites after 6–7 days. These
merozoites flood out into the blood and actively invade red
blood cells, taking only 20–30 s to do so. Within the circulating red blood cell the merozoite begins to feed on haemoglobin and transforms into a uninucleate feeding stage
called a trophozoite, shortly after which the nucleus begins
to divide and the parasite becomes a schizont. At this stage
the infected cells disappear from the circulation and adhere
to endothelial cells of various internal organs, a process
known as sequestration. Nuclear division occurs until about
16 merozoites are formed and these break out of the cell
and invade new circulating red blood cells. This process is

Figure 4.4
Schematic representation of the life cycle of a malaria parasite indicating points of immune attack and potential targets for immunological intervention.
(a) sporozoite in the blood, (b) initial invasion of hepatocyte, (c) early stage in the hepatocyte, (d) mature exoerythrocytic schizont (apparently not affected by immune response), (e) merozoite invasion of erythrocyte, (f) early erythrocytic form, (g) mature erythrocytic schizont, (h–m) mosquito stages. (After Cox, F.E.G., 1992, *Nature*, **360**, p. 471. Copyright Macmillan Magazines Ltd. For further information see the text.)

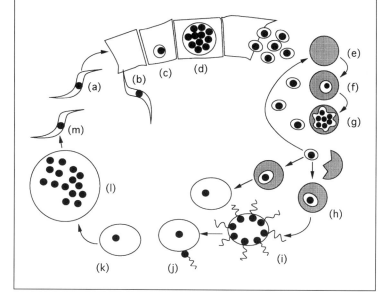

repeated almost indefinitely. The emergence of merozoites is accompanied by the release of toxic substances and the erythrocytic stages are responsible for the pathology associated with malaria. After a while some young merozoites develop into male and female gametocytes and these circulate in the peripheral blood until they are taken up by a mosquito when it feeds. Within the mosquito the gametocytes mature into male and female gametes, fertilization occurs, a zygote called an ookinete is formed and this is followed by another massive phase of multiplication resulting in the formation of sporozoites that migrate to the salivary glands to be injected when the mosquito feeds. The life cycles of the other malaria parasites of humans differ in the length of the exoerythrocytic and erythrocytic schizogonies, the numbers of merozoites produced and the absence of sequestration. Some strains of *P. vivax* have a persistent dormant exoerythrocytic phase.

Epidemiological studies have revealed that although some patients die, usually children or adults who have not been exposed before, malaria infections are long lived; individuals can be reinfected after natural recovery or cure and immunity gradually builds up over a period of years, fades quickly and is largely strain specific. Immunity to malaria is therefore the norm but is often incomplete and may take many years and numerous exposures to the bites of infected mosquitoes to develop. As in other parasitic infections, much of the information we have about immunity to malaria has been gleaned from laboratory studies, mainly in mice infected with rodent-derived species of *Plasmodium* and must, therefore, be regarded with caution. For further information see Hommel and Gilles (1998).

Malaria parasites are relatively free from immune attack when they are intracellular but are susceptible when the newly injected sporozoites circulate in the blood before reaching the liver, when merozoites are liberated from the liver into the bloodstream and before they invade red blood cells, and when merozoites have been released from red blood cells but before they invade new cells. Sporozoites are obvious targets for immune recognition and attack as they are free in the blood for 30–45 min before they penetrate liver cells. Sporozoites possess a highly immunogenic, immunodominant, 40–60 kDa protein surface coat, called the circumsporozoite protein (CSP), that in *P. falciparum* includes a dominant epitope consisting of four amino acids, asparagine–alanine–asparagine–proline repeated 37 times, written in the single letter code as $(NANP)_{37}$, and three or four copies of a smaller repeat, asparagine–valine–aspartate–proline (NVDP), dispersed throughout the CSP. Other species of malaria parasite have similar repeat regions but with different amino acid sequences. The repeat sequence of the CSP elicits a strong antibody response but, when exposed to antibody, the surface molecules cross-link enabling the sporozoite to shed its coat and thus escape from immune attack. The repeat sequence may, therefore, enable the parasites to evade the immune response by acting as a 'smoke screen' that deflects the response away from more susceptible targets. However, the sporozoite may still be a possible target for immune attack and current research is concentrating on the importance of antigens from the non-repeat regions of the CSP and those involved in the penetration of the liver hepatocytes.

Until recently it was assumed that once the malaria parasite had entered the liver hepatocytes there was no immune response as there are no signs of any significant inflammation or lymphocyte infiltration even when the exoerythrocytic schizont is fully mature. However, in murine malaria models there are a number of cell-mediated responses including a T_C-cell response to the early stages in the liver, targeted to parasite antigen(s) recognized in the context of liver cell MHC class I molecules, and also macrophage activation as evidenced by the production of IFN-γ, TNF and NO. Several liver stage antigens have now been identified and characterized and some of these share common epitopes with sporozoite antigens, for example LSA-1 (liver stage antigen-1). It is not clear what the actual mechanisms of immunity are or what happens in humans. In West Africa the outcome of infection is associated with certain MHC class I molecules, but there is less evidence that this is the case elsewhere.

The erythrocytic stages, particularly the merozoites, are obvious targets for attack (reviewed by Smith *et al.*, 1998). Several of the antigens involved have been characterized and cloned (Table 4.4). Like the sporozoite CSP molecule, many of these antigens are characterized by the presence of repeats of amino acids, raising the possibility that they could also be involved in immune evasion. In addition, many of the antigens identified exhibit considerable degrees of diversity and some even undergo antigenic variation (Reeder and Brown, 1996). This makes it very difficult for the host to mount an effective immune response and also explains why malaria infections persist for so long and why immunity does not build up until the host has experienced a wide range of antigens. Nevertheless, several erythrocytic stage antigens appear to play significant roles in immunity to malaria (reviewed by Howard and Pasloske, 1993; Facer and Tanner, 1997). Associated with the merozoite surface of all malaria parasites are a number of antigens including a 190–195 kDa glycoprotein, MSA-1, the merozoite surface antigen-1. Antibodies against MSA-1 block red blood cell invasion, so this could be a major target for immune attack. However, there is considerable diversity between isolates of MSA-1 and immunity to one isolate does not confer immunity to another. Other important merozoite antigens include AMA-1 (apical membrane antigen) associated with rhoptries (internal organelles involved in erythrocyte invasion) of the merozoite, RESA (ring-infected erythrocyte surface antigen) associated with merozoite dense granules, and EBA-175 (erythrocyte-binding antigen) associated with merozoite micronemes. All of these are involved in binding to or invading red blood cells and could be possible targets for immune attack. In addition there are a number of antigens associated with the membrane of infected erythrocytes, the

Table 4.4 Some *Plasmodium falciparum* candidate vaccines

Antigen	Location	Function
CS Circumsporozoite	Sporozoite and hepatocyte surface	Inhibition of hepatocyte invasion
TRAP (SSP-2) Thrombospondin-related anonymous protein	Sporozoite and hepatocyte surface	Inhibition of hepatocyte invasion
LSA-1 Liver stage antigen-1	Hepatocyte surface	NK
MSA-1 (MSP-1) Merozoite surface antigen-(protein-)1	Merozoite surface	Inhibition of erythrocyte invasion
MSA-2 (MSP-2) Merozoite surface antigen-(protein-)2	Merozoite surface	NK
RESA (Pf155) Ring-infected erythrocyte surface antigen	Merozoite dense granules	NK
EBA-175 Erythrocyte-binding antigen-175	Merozoite apical complex	Inhibition of erythrocyte invasion
AMA-1 Apical membrane antigen-1	Merozoite rhoptry	Inhibition of erythrocyte invasion
SPf66 Synthetic vaccine	Three merozoite antigens	NK
PfEMP-1 Erythrocyte membrane protein-1	Infected erythrocyte surface	Cytoadherence
SERA Serine-rich antigen	Released at schizogony	NK
Pfs25	Sexual stages	NK

This list is not complete but all the antigens listed have been tested on laboratory animals (mainly monkeys) with varying success. Further details are given in the text and by Facer and Tanner (1997).

most important of which is PfEMP-1 (*P. falciparum*-infected erythrocyte membrane protein-1). During the later schizogonic stages of *P. falciparum*, 'knobs' appear in the erythrocyte surface membrane and these are involved in adherence to endothelial cells and result in sequestration. The dominant molecule in these knobs is PfEMP-1, which is involved in both opsonization and agglutination of infected red blood cells. The actual role of PfEMP-1 is unclear but it is thought that sequestration prevents infected erythrocytes from circulating through the spleen, thus protecting them from the killing mechanisms that appear to operate there. Antibodies against PfEMP-1 prevent sequestration and facilitate parasite destruction in the spleen (see below).

The actual mechanisms whereby the host inhibits parasite replication are not clear. Antibody, specifically IgG, certainly plays a role in immunity to malaria as evidenced by the fact that the passive transfer of immune serum and maternal antibodies confer immunity in animals and humans. How antibody works is another question. Blocking of erythrocyte invasion is one obvious way but there are a number of other possibilities including agglutination of merozoites and infected cells and the involvement of macrophages in opsonization. Cell-mediated mechanisms, particularly the release of ROI, NO and TNF by macrophages, also appear to be involved in parasite killing. Where the destruction of parasites occurs is not known but it does not seem to be in the circulating blood. The most likely site is the spleen and evidence for this comes from experimental models and the fact that individuals who have had their spleens removed often suffer severe recrudescences of parasitaemia. What probably happens is that the flow of blood is slowed down in the spleen and the infected erythrocytes come in close contact with macrophages lining the blood vessels causing the release of ROI, NO and TNF that damage the intraerythrocytic parasites while infected cells and free merozoites are phagocytosed.

Several antigens are associated with gametocytes. Male and female gametes and zygotes are susceptible to antibody attack when taken up by a mosquito together with antibodies in the serum and are either killed or inactivated so that the infection in the mosquito cannot proceed. Antigens involved include a 250 kDa molecule on the gametocytes, gametes and zygotes, a 25 kDa molecule on the gametes and zygotes, and a 48 kDa molecule on the zygotes.

A major problem in the induction of immunity to malaria is that the various stages in the life cycle are morphologically, biochemically and antigenically distinct so, in effect, the infected person experiences a series of unrelated exposures to the same parasite. Thus immune responses to the sporozoite stage do not protect against the liver stage, immunity to the liver stage does not protect against the blood stages, and immunity to one isolate of the blood stages of the parasite is not effective against another. The acquisition of immunity, therefore, involves a number of components working together or in sequence. It is therefore impossible to implicate any particular mechanism in protective immunity

and it is likely that overall immunity results from a combination of a number of different responses and that there
may also be alternative mechanisms if one fails. All this
takes a long time and, as a consequence, there are numerous
opportunities for something to go wrong and one result is
that much of the pathology of malaria reflects the adverse
side effects of the protective immune response. For example,
some of the symptoms of cerebral malaria are caused by
macrophage products such as ROI, NO and TNF elicited as
part of the immune response, which may cause blockage
and sludging of capillaries or affect the signalling pathways
in the brain leading to coma and other cerebral symptoms
as well as causing direct damage to the parasites themselves
(see Clark and Rockett, 1996; Grau, 1996). Macrophage products are also probably involved in the hypoglycaemia and
anaemia associated with malaria. This knowledge is beginning to pinpoint ways of halting or reversing adverse reactions, for example TNF contributes to the production of NO
and anti-TNF has been used to treat children with cerebral
malaria. Another approach is to target the toxins released
when the infected red cells in the blood rupture.

This brings us on to the possibility of a vaccine against
malaria. The control of malaria is one of the most pressing
needs in tropical countries at the present time. However,
there are insufficient tools at our disposal as resistance has
developed against the most effective drug, chloroquine, there
are few new drugs in development and anti-mosquito measures have become less effective as insecticide resistance has
spread worldwide. The control of malaria would be facilitated if a vaccine against malaria was available and the
possibility of developing one has attracted a vast amount of
effort. However, despite the fact that it has cost many millions of dollars, we still do not have a vaccine. Theoretically
a vaccine against malaria should be possible for a number
of reasons. First, most people do recover and, out of the 350
million or so infected, fewer than 2–3 million die and most
of those that do recover subsequently develop some resistance. Secondly, numerous animal experiments have proved
that it is possible to induce some degree of protection artifi-
cially and this has given scientists hope that this might also
happen in humans. There are problems, however, and these
are: (i) immunity is slow to develop and often incomplete
in that infections in recovered individuals do occur although
they are less life-threatening; (ii) immunity is usually specific to local strains of the parasite; and (iii) experimental
immunization is rarely completely successful and often
involves the use of methods of vaccination that would be

unacceptable for human use. The aim, therefore, must be to develop a vaccine that is better than natural immunity. This is a major challenge that must take into consideration what stage of the life cycle of the parasite to attack and what kind of antigens to use. The major problem is that, as pointed out above, the malaria life cycle is very complex and includes a number of biochemically and immunologically distinct stages.

The current approach is to identify and characterize potentially protective surface antigens and to use these as subunit antigens on their own, as recombinant molecules expressed in a suitable vector or as a basis for synthetic vaccines. All three methods have been tried with varying success as have experimental DNA vaccines (reviewed by Jones and Hoffman, 1994; Hoffman, 1996; Facer and Tanner, 1997).

All stages of the life cycle must be regarded as possible targets and each must be approached separately. Sporozoites are obvious targets as they are the first stages to enter the body and circulate in the blood for a short time before entering the liver. A vaccine against the sporozoite would prevent infection and early experiments showed that immunization with irradiated sporozoites did protect mice and was partly protective in humans. The repeat region of the circumsporozoite protein of the sporozoite (NANP) has been used as a basis for recombinant and synthetic vaccines. Early trials were promising and indicated an efficacy of about 20 per cent, but also revealed that there was little correlation between antibody levels to NANP and protection. It is now widely accepted that the sporozoite repeat antigen is not a good vaccine candidate and a number of other sporozoite antigens from outside the repeat region are currently receiving attention.

Liver stages are also possible vaccination targets. Although several liver stage antigens that are possible targets for immune attack, including LSA-1, have been recognized, there is currently no vaccine under development.

Blood stages are obvious targets because there are so many of them and because they cause the disease. A number of potential antigens have been recognized either associated with the infected red cell, intraerythrocytic parasites or merozoites, or with secreted molecules. Several *P. falciparum* antigens are currently being considered as candidate vaccines. MSA-1 involved in invasion of red cells by merozoites is currently undergoing safety and efficacy trials. Other molecules scheduled for trials include AMA-1, also involved in red cell invasion, and EBA-175, a merozoite antigen involved in binding to red blood cells and blocking red cell invasion. SERA (serine-rich antigen), released when the schizont bursts, is protective in monkeys although it is not known how this happens, but field trials are currently being planned.

The only vaccine that has undergone extensive field trials is SPf66 developed by the Colombian biochemist, Manuel Patarroyo (see Targett, 1995; Facer and Tanner, 1997). This is a synthetic vaccine consisting of a polymer of three merozoite antigens linked by the sporozoite antigen NANP. The three components are Pf83, an 83 kDa peptide representing part of MSA-1, Pf55 and Pf35, none of which has been identified with any of the known major malaria antigens. This vaccine was developed following extensive trials of various peptides in owl monkeys belonging to the genus *Aotus* and has now been tested in *Aotus* monkeys and in humans. The first human trials involved safety and immunogenicity in over 15 000 individuals in the Tumaco region of Colombia where malaria is present and the next involved 751 soldiers in the same area. These trials showed that the vaccine was safe and immunogenic and, although it did not prevent malaria, it reduced the number of malaria episodes significantly. This vaccine was subsequently approved by the WHO and underwent more extensive trials in natural populations of adults and children in South America, Africa and Thailand. The results of these trials have been promising but also discouraging. In all those vaccinated, the vaccine is immunogenic and well tolerated. On the other hand, the vaccine does not prevent malaria although, in areas of more intense transmission, it does appear to reduce the number of episodes but to a lesser extent than in the initial trials. However, assessing these results tends to be subjective and, in the past, there has been a tendency to interpret the results overoptimistically. The major problem, however, is that the vaccine seems to be least effective in the most susceptible groups, young children in regions such as The Gambia where transmission is intense and where the vaccine is most needed. It is probably too early to say whether or not SPf66 has a future, but it can be regarded as a first-generation vaccine and represents a change of approach towards reducing the burden of malaria and the number of episodes rather than trying to prevent infection altogether. It also depends on repeated reinfection in order to boost the immunity, thus the more people are exposed to infection, the stronger their immunity becomes.

The only other vaccines currently being considered are ones that target the sexual stages in the mosquito. At first this might seem to be an irrational approach but it is both logical and feasible. In the mosquito gut, the sexual stages emerge from the red blood cells and are recognized by antibodies taken up in the same blood meal. The principle of this vaccine is to immunize individuals with sexual stage antigens in order to raise antibodies which will inactivate these stages when taken up by a mosquito. This transmission-blocking vaccine has been called 'altruistic' because it does not protect the person immunized although it does prevent transmission. Pfs25, an antigen on the surface of the malaria zygote, is the most favoured candidate for a vaccine and safety and efficacy trials are underway. Until recently, the idea of such a vaccine would have been unthinkable, but if current opinion favours a vaccine that reduces the burden of malaria without actually preventing it, there is no reason why such a transmission-blocking antigen should not be added to SPf66 as a 'cocktail'.

Numerous other possibilities are currently being pursued and it will probably be necessary to have a multipronged approach (see Hoffman, 1996). Once the concept of a cocktail vaccine that does not necessarily produce sterile immunity but does reduce the severity of the infection has been accepted, it might be worth considering novel approaches such as vaccinating against disease. Laboratory animals have been vaccinated against the toxins produced by the malaria parasite and antibodies against TNF have been shown to be beneficial in ameliorating the severity of human cerebral malaria. Other approaches still at the experimental stage involve the use of antigens expressed in viruses or bacteria or incorporated into DNA vaccines. In order to mimic the multistage immunity that is thought to occur in malaria, there has recently been a trend towards the use of multiple antigen peptides incorporating T- and B-cell epitopes and a number of malaria antigens from different stages in the life cycle (see Doolan and Hoffman, 1997). Some of these multivalent vaccines are now undergoing experimental trials either as synthetic molecules or as DNA vaccines. One such vaccine incorporates several antigens including CSP, LSA-1, MSA-1, AMA-1 and Pfs25 (see Facer and Tanner, 1997).

4.5 Immunity to parasitic helminths

Infections with helminth worms tend to be long and chronic and the burden of infection depends on the number of infected stages ingested or introduced through the skin. In the examples considered in this chapter, the infective stages are larvae that are structurally and antigenically different from the adults into which they eventually develop. The size of adult and larval helminth worms means that they cannot easily be attacked by antibodies or phagocytosed. ADCC (see Chapter 1), often involving eosinophils as well as macrophages, is one of the main mechanisms whereby immunity is effected and is therefore predominantly of the T_H2 type although there is increasing evidence of T_H1-cell involvement. Most adult helminth parasites have evolved ways of evading the immune response and also generating immune responses that are effective against larval stages of the same species. Protective immune responses are, therefore, usually targeted against newly arrived larval stages, a phenomenon known as concomitant immunity, which soon fades after the adult worms die or are removed. From an evolutionary point of view, this mechanism serves to limit the parasite burden and is an example of one of the ways in which a parasite can manipulate the immune system in order to favour its own survival. However, in humans the combination of long infections and the continual mounting of immune responses often leads to immunopathological damage which, in most cases, is more serious than the infection caused by the worms themselves (see Riffkin *et al.*, 1996; Freedman, 1997).

4.5.1 *Immunology of schistosomiasis*

Schistosomiasis is caused by infection with helminth worms belonging to the genus *Schistosoma*. Humans are infected with several species of which the most important are *S. mansoni*, *S. japonicum* and *S. haematobium*. These are large worms, 15–20 mm in length, that live in the lumen of blood vessels associated with the intestine or bladder in the case of *S. haematobium*. Schistosomes have complex life cycles alternating between the human host and a snail. The infection in humans begins when free swimming schistosome larvae called cercariae penetrate the skin, where they develop into the next larval stages, schistosomula. These remain in the skin for 3–4 days before being carried in the bloodstream first to the lungs, then to the portal system and finally to sites in mesenteric or bladder blood vessels. Here the worms mature into males and females that pair for life and attach to the walls of the blood vessel where they may live for 5 years or more. During this time the female worm produces millions of eggs, some of which are passed out in the faeces or urine into freshwater. Here the eggs hatch releasing a ciliated larva called a miracidium that finds and invades a suitable snail within which two generations of multiplication occur culminating in the production of large numbers of cercariae larvae that emerge and infect a new victim. Each stage in the life cycle is characterized by massive morphological, physiological and biochemical changes which have major implications for the immune system of the human host. For further information see Kojima (1998).

Immunity to schistosomiasis is slow to develop and at one time it was thought that humans did not develop any immunity and that the decline in prevalence seen in individuals over the age of about 15 years in epidemiological studies represented reductions in exposure to infection rather than the acquisition of immunity. However, as a result of extensive observations on populations who were continually monitored after exposure to infection and drug treatment, it is now known that immunity to schistosomiasis does occur and there is also evidence from laboratory studies that this is the case (see Pearce, 1995). Most of what we know has come from studies on *S. mansoni* and, unless stated otherwise, everything that follows relates to this parasite although there are a few significant differences in the immune response to different species of schistosomes.

As in malaria, there are two aspects of immunity that must be considered, recovery from an initial infection and prevention of reinfection. In order to understand these two aspects a more detailed analysis of the life cycle must be undertaken. On penetrating the host's skin the surfaces of the cercariae undergo massive adaptive changes that enable the worms to transform from aquatic larvae into parasitic schistosomula. Part of the outer surface, or tegument, is shed and a new tegument acquired. This tegument is a very active structure and has the ability to absorb a range of host molecules including red blood cell A and B glycolipids, immunoglobulins, complement components and MHC molecules. These effectively disguise the worm as its host, thus it is able to travel through the body and to remain in its final immunologically exposed site unrecognized. However, the worm produces a number of secretions and excretions that are immunogenic and elicit appropriate antibody responses. In addition, many of the eggs produced by the female worm do not reach the outside world; some are deposited locally and some are carried around the body and deposited in the liver. These eggs produce a number of highly immunogenic molecules, known as soluble egg antigens (SEA), that pass out through pores in the egg and these also elicit immune responses. Some of the antigens are common to the egg, larva and adult worm. The net result is that the host mounts a series of immune responses that are ineffective against the disguised adult worms but are effective against subsequent invading larvae, the phenomenon of concomitant immunity. However, there is a down side to this because the eggs in the tissues are also recognized as foreign and the immune responses elicited bring about the formation of granulomas resulting in gross pathological changes to the liver and increased portal blood pressure, which are major causes of morbidity and mortality in schistosomiasis. Similarly, eggs deposited in the bladder eventually lead to immunologically mediated calcification.

There is some evidence of immunity to a primary infection although relatively little is known about the actual events involved. Egg production is inhibited by antibodies, some presumably generated against eggs and some against an antigen known as Sm28-GST (see below). The parasite also seems to be able to manipulate the immune response and, during the course of an infection, there is a switch from T_H1- to T_H2-type responses. It is interesting to note that egg production is actually enhanced by TNF, so if the activation of macrophages is inhibited and TNF production reduced, this switch to T_H2-type responses would actually reduce fecundity. This could be a mechanism employed by the host to reduce the possibility of damage caused by schistosome eggs and is another example of cross-regulation between T_H1 and T_H2 cytokines in parasitic infections. Overall, however, antibodies play only a minor role in controlling an ongoing infection.

Immunity to a second or subsequent challenge is another matter and the newly arrived larvae are extremely vulnerable to immune attack once they have shed their coats and before they have acquired any host antigens. Much of what we know about these events has been derived from laboratory studies but a number of realistic extrapolations to humans can be made. Immune attack at this stage is multifactorial and involves ADCC. The actual mechanisms vary from host to host but the two major players are IgE and eosinophils, and IgG or IgE and macrophages. IgE binds to the schistosomulum and the eosinophil flattens out along the larval worm and releases a substance called major basic protein (MBP) on to the worm's surface. This disrupts the tegument and allows the eosinophil to penetrate under and strip off the tegument causing the death of the worm. Macrophages also bind to the worm via IgG and release toxic molecules, including NO, on to the surface of the worm, facilitating its destruction. A number of other mechanisms, some involving neutrophils and platelets and complement-mediated killing, have also been implicated but not IFN-γ or

T_C-cell killing, thus the protective immune response is essentially of the T_H2 cell type. There is some controversy concerning the actual site where the larval worms are killed, some observers suggest that it is in the skin and others that it is in the lungs, a proposition that is gaining support (see Coulson, 1997; Mountford and Harrop, 1998).

The pathology of schistosomiasis is largely associated with eggs deposited in the liver around which a granuloma forms. At one time it was thought that the granuloma represented a T_H1 cell-mediated DTH reaction, but it is now known that the cells involved are actually eosinophils and the antibody is IgE, thus the cytokines involved include T_H2 cell products. It is possible that in schistosomiasis the T_H1 mechanisms are actually anti-inflammatory as IL-12, which drives the immune response towards the T_H1 pole, is involved in the regression of granulomas and prevents their formation.

Vaccination against schistosomiasis is a realistic possibility (reviewed by Berquist and Colley, 1998) and in theory all that is necessary is to bypass the primary infection and to induce an immune response that is effective against newly invading cercariae. There is considerable evidence that this can be done from experimental models, for example irradiated, but not killed, cercariae induce a strong immunity and this method has been used to protect cattle against *Schistosoma mattheei*. This would not, of course, be possible against human schistosomes, but these results have encouraged the selection of a number of candidate molecules, some of which are currently undergoing trials for safety and immunogenicity. These include paramyosin, a muscle protein found only in invertebrates, and two schistosome enzymes, glutathione-*S*-transferase (GST) and triose phosphate isomerase (TPI) (see Table 4.5). It must be borne in mind, however, that the maximum efficacy so far achieved in animal models is 30–80 per cent and optimistic estimates of the maximum likely to be achieved is in the range of 80–90 per cent, so any vaccine is unlikely to be the panacea for schistosomiasis. There is, however, a case for an anti-disease vaccine that would prevent morbidity but not infection and such a vaccine might be targeted against the development of granulomas; experimentally, the use of egg antigens plus IL-12, which drives the immune response towards the T_H1 pole, has been encouraging (Wynn *et al.*, 1995). A vaccine that reduced the fecundity of the female worms might also help to reduce pathology. In spite of the amount of interest in developing a vaccine against schistosomiasis, it must be pointed out that there are several very effective drugs in use, particularly praziquantel, and that anti-snail measures have also been very successful.

Table 4.5 Some *Schistosoma mansoni* candidate vaccines

Antigen	Nature of antigen
Glutathione-*S*-transferase (GST)	Enzyme Adults and schistosomula
Paramyosin (Sm97)	Invertebrate muscle protein Adults and schistosomula
Irradiated vaccine antigen-5 (IrV-5)	Vertebrate muscle protein All stages
MAP-3 (Sm23)	Synthetic peptide from integral membrane protein All stages
MAP-4 (TPI)	Synthetic peptide from triose phosphate isomerase All stages

All these antigens have been tested on mice and GST and IrV-5 have also been tested on rats and baboons with protection rates ranging from 25–60%. GST, Sm97 and MAP-3 are undergoing phase I (safety and immunogenicity) trials. IrV-5 and MAP-4 are being considered as DNA constructs. (Source: WHO *TDR News*, No. 54, October 1997.)

4.5.2 *Immunology of filariasis*

Human filariasis is caused by infections with a number of species of nematode worms, the females of which produce larvae that are released in the body of the host, often in the blood, until taken up by an arthropod vector. The most important manifestations are lymphatic filariasis and onchocerciasis. In lymphatic filariasis, caused by *Wuchereria bancrofti*, *Brugia malayi* and *Brugia timori* and transmitted by mosquitoes, the adults live in the lymphatic system and the disease is characterized by lymphatic blockage resulting in gross swelling of the limbs, scrotum and other parts of the body causing the condition known as elephantiasis. In onchocerciasis, caused by *Onchocerca volvulus* and transmitted by blackflies belonging to the genus *Simulium*, the adults live in skin nodules and the disease is characterized by blindness. The life cycles are basically similar. The infection begins when infective third-stage larvae are deposited on the skin by the insect vector when it feeds. The larvae enter the body via the bite, migrate around the body, grow, moult and mature into male and female adults which mate. The female produces first-stage larvae, known as microfilariae, that are subsequently taken up by the insect vector within which two further moults occur, resulting in the production of infective third-stage larvae that, when introduced into a fresh host, initiate a new infection. The immunology and pathology of lymphatic filariasis and onchocerciasis are sufficiently different to justify separate consideration.

Lymphatic filariasis

Lymphatic filariasis comprises a spectrum of disease; some individuals show no signs of infection, others have high levels of microfilariae in their blood (microfilaraemia) but few signs of disease, and others harbour few microfilariae but exhibit marked pathological changes. Adult worms in the lymphatic system are very long lived, 10 years or more, which suggests that there is very little immunity to primary infections. However, during her lifetime the female produces millions of microfilariae, all capable of eliciting immune responses and many of which die. As a working hypothesis it seems that the worms of the primary infection do not evoke an immune response and that any immunity generated is directed against microfilariae and newly invading larvae that are antigenically different from the microfilariae in the blood. There are few laboratory models for filariasis and those that do exist are not entirely satisfactory, thus very little is known about the actual mechanisms of immunity and immunopathology but what is known is soundly based on observations on human infections. For further information see Muller and Wakelin (1998).

Several clues about the nature of the immune response can be obtained from detailed considerations of the patterns of infections in different individuals who exhibit a range of clinical manifestations. As mentioned above, some individuals have no microfilariae and no pathology despite intensive exposure to infection in endemic areas. These people, known as 'endemic normals', show no signs of any acquired immune responses although their T cells are capable of responding to filarial antigens, suggesting that they have been exposed to infection. Whether or not this means that they are inherently non-susceptible is unclear. Most infected individuals harbour large numbers of microfilariae but show no obvious signs of pathology; their immune systems are hyporesponsive, they have low levels of specific antibodies, poor cell-mediated responses and are unable to clear their parasitaemias. The third category contains individuals harbouring few microfilariae but exhibiting severe pathological changes as indicated by lymphatic blockage (elephantiasis), fever and other symptoms. In these individuals, both antibody and cell-mediated immune responses are elevated. A fourth category contains individuals with high levels

of eosinophils and exaggerated IgE responses, a condition
known as tropical pulmonary eosinophilia (TPE). Epidemiological studies indicate that there is a good correlation
between the clearance of parasites and the development of
pathological changes and that this is age related. This suggests that pathology may be associated with an ongoing
immune response characterized by an increase in eosinophilia and IgE. However, this transition from infected but
asymptomatic to uninfected but symptomatic does not always
occur.

Overall, overt lymphatic filariasis is characterized by a
period of immune hyporesponsiveness and anergy to filarial antigens and a down-regulation of antibody production,
followed by a return to responsiveness accompanied by the
progressive development of obstructive lesions leading to
elephantiasis. Little is known about the mechanisms underlying the initial immunosuppression that enhances the survival of the first generation of worms. Filarial antigens appear
to be involved in the induction of hyporesponsiveness as
evidenced by the fact that prenatal exposure to such antigens leads to higher levels of microfilaraemia, suggesting
the induction of a parasite-induced state of tolerance which,
however, is reversible.

As the infection progresses IgE and IgG4 levels, both
targeted at the same antigens, rise and the amounts of IgG4
become exceptionally high. The return to immune responsiveness is also accompanied by increases in the levels of
IgG1, IgG2 and IgG3 and progressive chronic pathological
changes (see Maizels *et al.*, 1995).

During the course of an infection the adult worms in the
lymphatic system remain unaffected by the immune response, but some protective immunity is developed directed
against the microfilariae in the blood or larvae introduced
by a mosquito. Evidence that this occurs comes from experiments in which irradiated larvae have been shown to induce protective immune responses in laboratory animals.
The cuticle of filarial larvae is very thin compared with that
of intestinal nematodes and possesses a number of possible targets for immunological attack, but only a few of
the molecules involved have been properly characterized.
Experimentally, the most commonly demonstrated killing
mechanism is ADCC involving IgG, IgE, eosinophils, macrophages and neutrophils. These cells adhere to the surface of
the larva via an antibody bridge and secrete toxic substances
on to the surface of the worm. As well as the surface antigens, a number of internal antigens have also been incriminated as possible targets and these include paramyosin which

has been shown to be a protective antigen in schistosomiasis. The most important antibodies involved in protection are IgE. This suggests that immunity to microfilariae is essentially antibody-mediated and is, therefore, of the T_H2 type. There is, however, a further complication in that while IgE is thought to be protective, IgG may be counterprotective by blocking possible IgE-binding sites. It must also be pointed out that humans infected with *Brugia malayi* show a correlation between T_H1 responses and low levels of infection suggesting a protective role for cell-mediated responses and the involvement of IFN-γ.

Other antibodies, IgG1, IgG2 and IgG3, are involved in pathology and, of these, IgG3 may be the most important as it is implicated in type III immune complex-mediated hypersensitivity reactions which could result in the kind of destructive lesions seen in elephantiasis. The source of the antigens involved is not known but there are abundant microfilarial antigens in the blood.

In summary, all the evidence available suggests that the filarial worms are able to manipulate the immune response in order to enhance their own survival and to establish a state of concomitant immunity which may later backfire as immunopathological processes are generated, as has been described in schistosomiasis. As in schistosomiasis, filarial worms are caught up in the complex network of cytokine regulation and cross-regulation of the immune response which changes during the course of the infection and as yet we do not really understand what is actually responsible for immunity and what is involved in immunopathology. Also, as in other parasitic infections, the dichotomy between T_H1 and T_H2 responses is not as clear as it was once thought to be (see Nutman, 1995).

Against this background, vaccination against lymphatic filariasis is not a realistic possibility given that the majority of people infected do not suffer any adverse effects and that severe pathology is probably immunologically mediated. In any case, there are good, cheap and effective drugs against both the adult worms and microfilariae.

Onchocerciasis

Onchocerciasis, which has many features in common with lymphatic filariasis, is caused by infection with the filarial nematode *Onchocerca volvulus* transmitted by the black-flies belonging to the genus *Simulium*. The infective larvae moult twice and mature to adults in subcutaneous connective tissue, muscle or fibrous nodules which may contain several worms. The adult worms live for 9–14 years and the females produce microfilariae at a rate of 700–1500 per day. Many do not survive but those that do migrate to the skin, eyes and other organs and have a lifespan of 6–24 months. Like lymphatic filariasis, onchocerciasis represents a spectrum of disease states; most infected individuals are asymptomatic but others suffer from damage to the skin, eyes and lymphatic system. The eye lesions include sclerosing keratitis and damage to the optic nerve resulting in progressive loss of vision and blindness. For further information see Whitworth (1998).

There are no good animal models of onchocerciasis so our knowledge of the immunology of the disease is fragmentary. However, there are similarities with lymphatic filariasis and a number of parallels can be drawn. At one pole are the majority, the 'endemic normals', who are apparently uninfected, then there are those who harbour large numbers of microfilariae but who are hyporesponsive and, at the other pole, are those exhibiting considerable signs of pathology. The 'endemic normals' may well have some innate immunity. Hyporesponsiveness is specific so is presumably generated by worm antigens. Over a period of 1–2 years after infection a number of immunological changes occur. In some individuals there is no return to immune responsiveness, whereas in others there is and this is accompanied by a rise in the levels of IgG and IgE. During the period of restored immune responsiveness, neither the living adults nor the microfilariae seem to be adversely affected although, in experimental models, eosinophils can be seen to adhere to microfilariae. On the other hand, dead parasites evoke strong immune responses and these constitute the basis of the pathology associated with this infection. Local reactions include lymphocyte-mediated inflammation around dead adults in the nodules and microfilariae in the skin and eyes. Various immune mechanisms have been implicated in the pathology including immediate sensitivity type I reactions involving IgE, type III immune complex reactions involving IgG and type IV antibody-independent cell-mediated responses. Autoantibodies against ocular tissues are also produced. The most severe skin reactions are associated with the condition known as sowda, a localized dermatitis in which considerable areas of the skin becomes swollen and the associated lymph nodes greatly enlarged. Sowda is correlated with high levels of antibody and few microfilariae in the lesions themselves. It is still an open question as to whether the misdirected immune responses are caused by the death of the worms and the release of internal antigens or whether the immune response actually kills the worms.

The fact that treatment with the drug diethylcarbamazine is often accompanied by strong skin reactions, called Mazzotti reactions, supports the first hypothesis.

The possible adverse effects of treatment with diethylcarbamazine have been circumvented by more recent chemotherapy, particularly the very effective microfilaricide, ivermectin, which is well tolerated and is the mainstay of current control programmes. Indeed, the WHO confidently predicts the eradication of onchocerciasis, so in the long term there is no need for a vaccine.

4.6   Parasitic infections and AIDS

The spread of HIV and AIDS throughout much of the tropics has had a marked effect on the control of parasitic infections as much of the money required for the development of anti-parasitic measures has been diverted to research on AIDS. Although HIV constitutes a major health risk, the numbers infected (30 million) represent only a fraction of those infected with parasites and this disproportionate funding is bound to affect the development of vaccines against parasitic diseases. The second problem is that there are increasing numbers of individuals co-infected with HIV and parasites. Fortunately, the situation is not as bad as it might be with respect to the major parasitic infections discussed in this chapter; there is no evidence that malaria and HIV affect one another and there have only been a few recorded cases of any interactions in Chagas' disease, African trypanosomiasis, schistosomiasis, filariasis or onchocerciasis. On the other hand, co-infection with visceral leishmaniasis and HIV has been recorded, particularly in southern Europe, Brazil and East Africa, but the incidence is increasing elsewhere to such an extent that the WHO now recognizes this co-infection as an emerging disease. The immunological basis of this particular interaction has yet to be resolved. The fact that the immunosuppression caused by HIV does not affect most parasites suggests that immunity to parasites is more firmly rooted than it initially appears to be. A number of other parasitic infections recrudesce or are enhanced in patients with AIDS and these include *Toxoplasma gondii*, *Cryptosporidium parvum*, *Isospora belli*, *Cyclospora cayetanensis* and the helminth worm *Strongyloides stercoralis*. In addition, several species of microsporidians have only been recorded from patients with AIDS. In conclusion, it can safely be assumed that the study of immunity to parasites can tell us something about the immune responses to HIV and vice versa.

Summary

- Parasitic infections caused by protozoa and helminth worms represent a threat to human health worldwide, but particularly in the tropics and subtropics where five diseases, leishmaniasis, African and South American trypanosomiasis, malaria, schistosomiasis and filariasis, predominate. These infections are characteristically long and chronic and accompanied by immunological dysfunction. This is because the infectious agents have evolved ways of evading the immune response and the result is that the immune responses are multifactorial and complex and in most cases become misdirected and damage the host instead of the parasite.

- Leishmaniasis is a disease caused by over 20 different species of *Leishmania*. These are intracellular parasites that are adapted to living within the phagolysosomes of macrophages. Much has been learned from the mouse model, *L. major*. The major form of immunity is mediated by T_H1 cells which activate infected macrophages to kill their intracellular parasites, mainly through the action of NO. Mouse strains that preferentially elicit T_H1 responses are therefore generally resistant to infection, whereas those that elicit T_H2 responses are susceptible.

- Trypanosomiasis is caused by *Trypanosoma* species. *T. cruzi*, the causative agent of New World trypanosomiasis, is a predominantly intracellular pathogen that resides mainly in macrophages and survives by erupting from the phagolysosome into the cytosol. The main form of immunity is mediated by macrophage activation. Blood-borne stages survive in part by being resistant to complement, and by expressing molecules that mimic host proteins to evade recognition. Antibodies elicited to these antigens cross-react with host antigens leading to autoimmune pathologies, particularly in cardiac muscle. *T. brucei* causes African trypanosomiasis (sleeping sickness). This organism is predominantly blood-borne and continually uses antigenic variation of a thick coat comprising variable surface glycoprotein (VSG) in order to evade developing antibody responses. Infections are therefore characterized with waves of blood parasitaemia as each new variant emerges. Both trypanosome species also induce generalized immunosuppression.

- Malaria is caused by several species of *Plasmodium* that are transmitted by mosquitoes. The most dangerous to humans is *P. falciparum*, although each is characterized by a complex life cycle comprising both intracellular (hepatocyte and erythrocyte) and blood-borne stages. In the blood the sporozoites are surrounded by circumsporozite protein (CSP). CSP is immunogenic although antibodies that bind cause shedding of CSP which helps protect the organism. Intrahepatocyte schizonts are susceptible to cytotoxic T lymphocytes, in which liver stage antigen-1 (LSA-1) appears to be a major antigen recognized.

- Helminth worms are too large to be ingested by phagocytic cells and remain extracellular. The main form of defence against these organisms is antibody-dependent cell-mediated cytotoxicity (ADCC). Schistosomiasis is a disease caused by three different species of *Schistosoma*, although *S. mansoni* is the best understood. Parasites invade as motile cercariae which are vulnerable to ADCC triggered by antibodies (particularly IgE) elicited by previous *Schistosoma* infections. These shed their coat to become schistosomula which take up residence in the blood vessels of the intestines and bladder.

Schistosomula are protected by acquiring a coat of host antigens which disguises them from the immune system; however, parasite antigens are secreted which elicit antibodies and which protect from subsequent infection. Pathology is caused by parasite eggs that become deposited in the liver and which cause granulomas. Filariasis is another helminth disease, which is actually a spectrum of diseases. Lymphatic filariasis is caused by *Wuchereria* and *Brugia* species in the lymphatic system which cause swelling (elephantiasis). Infection with these worms causes generalized immunosuppression although the mechanisms are not well understood. Onchocerciasis is caused by *Onchocerca volvulus* which lives in connective tissues liberating prodigious numbers of microfilariae. These disperse and can cause inflammatory damage to the skin, eyes and lymphatic system. Owing to the lack of an animal model, our understanding of the immunology to *Onchocerca* is fragmentary.

Study problems

1. 'In parasitic infections it is the immune response that causes the disease not the parasite itself.' What is the evidence for this statement?
2. Compare the ways in which *Leishmania*, *Trypanosoma* and *Plasmodium* evade the host's immune response.
3. Compare the efficacy of the immune responses to each of the stages in the life cycle of the malaria parasite.
4. How has *Leishmania* contributed to our understanding of how different T-helper subsets are involved in immunity to intracellular microorganisms?

Selected reading

Allen, J.E. and Maizels, R.M., 1997, T_H1–T_H2: reliable paradigm or dangerous dogma, *Immunol. Today*, **18**, 387–392

Ashford, R.W. and Bates, P.A., 1998, Leishmaniasis in the Old World, in Cox, F.E.G., Kreier, J.P. and Wakelin, D. (eds) *Topley and Wilson's Microbiology and Microbial Infections*, 9th edn, Vol. 5, *Parasitology*, London: Edward Arnold, pp. 215–240

Barry, J.D., 1997, The relative significance of mechanisms of antigenic variation in African trypanosomes, *Parasitol. Today*, **13**, 212–218

Berquist, R. and Colley, D., 1998, Schistosomiasis vaccines: research to development, *Parasitol. Today*, **14**, 99–104

Clark, I.A. and Rockett, K., 1996, Nitric oxide and parasitic disease, *Adv. Parasitol.*, **37**, 1–56

Constant, S.L. and Bottomly, K., 1997, Induction of T_H1 and T_H2 CD4$^+$ T cell responses: the alternative approaches, *Annu. Rev. Immunol.*, **15**, 297–322

Coulson, P., 1997, The radiation attenuated vaccine against schistosomiasis in animal models; paradigm for human vaccine, *Adv. Parasitol.*, **39**, 271–336

Cox, F.E.G., 1998, Classification of the parasitic protozoa, in Cox, F.E.G., Kreier, J.P and Wakelin, D. (eds) *Topley and Wilson's Microbiology and Microbial Infections*, 9th edn, Vol. 5, *Parasitology*, London: Edward Arnold, pp. 141–155

Cox, F.E.G. and Liew, F.Y., 1992, T-cell subsets and cytokines in parasitic infections, *Immunol. Today*, **13**, 445–448

Cox, F.E.G. and Wakelin, D., 1998, Immunology and immunopathology of human parasitic infections, in Cox, F.E.G., Kreier, J.P. and Wakelin, D. (eds) *Topley and Wilson's Microbiology and Microbial Infections*, 9th edn, Vol. 5, *Parasitology*, London: Edward Arnold, pp. 58–84

Doolan, D.L. and Hoffman, S.L., 1997, Multi-gene vaccination against malaria: a multistage, multi-immune response approach, *Parasitol. Today*, **13**, 171–178

DosReis, G.A., 1997, Cell-mediated immunity in experimental *Trypanosoma cruzi* infection, *Parasitol. Today*, **13**, 335–342

Facer, C.A. and Tanner, M., 1997, Clinical trials of malaria vaccines: progress and prospects, *Adv. Parasitol.*, **39**, 2–68

Freedman, D.O. (ed.), 1997, *Immunopathogenic Aspects of Disease Induced by Helminth Parasites, Chemical Immunology*, **66**, Basel: Karger

Gibson, D.I., 1998, Nature and classification of the parasitic helminths, in Cox, F.E G., Kreier, J.P. and Wakelin, D. (eds) *Topley and Wilson's Microbiology and Microbial*

Infections, 9th edn, Vol. 5, *Parasitology*, London: Edward Arnold, pp. 453–477

Grau, G.E., 1996, T-cell subsets and effector mechanisms of pathology in cerebral malaria, in Mustafa, A.S., Al-Attiyah, R.J., Nath, I. and Chugh, T.D. (eds) *T-Cell Subsets and Cytokine Interplay in Infectious Diseases*, Basel: Karger, pp. 63–71

Handman, E., 1997, *Leishmania* vaccines: old and new, *Parasitol. Today*, **13**, 236–238

Hoffman, S. (ed.), 1996, *Malaria Vaccine Development: a Multi-Immune Response Approach*, Washington: ASM Press

Hommel, M. and Gilles, H.M., 1998, Malaria, in Cox, F.E.G., Kreier, J.P. and Wakelin, D. (eds) *Topley and Wilson's Microbiology and Microbial Infections*, 9th edn, Vol. 5, *Parasitology*, London: Edward Arnold, pp. 362–409

Howard, R.J. and Pasloske, B.L., 1993, Target antigens for asexual malaria vaccine development, *Parasitol. Today*, **9**, 369–372

James, S.L., 1995, Role of nitric oxide in parasitic infections, *Microbiol. Rev.*, **59**, 533–547

Jones, T.R. and Hoffman, S.L., 1994. Malaria vaccine development, *Clin. Microbiol. Rev.*, **7**, 303–310

Kemp, M., Theander, T.G. and Kharazmi, A., 1996, The contrasting roles of CD4+ T cells in intracellular infections in humans: leishmaniasis as an example, *Immunol. Today*, **17**, 13–16

Kojima, S., 1998, Schistosomes, in Cox, F.E.G., Kreier, J.P. and Wakelin, D. (eds) *Topley and Wilson's Microbiology and Microbial Infections*, 9th edn, Vol. 5, *Parasitology*, London: Edward Arnold, pp. 479–505

Liew, F.Y. and O'Donnell, C.A., 1993, Immunology of leishmaniasis, *Adv. Parasitol.*, **32**, 161–181

MacMicking, J., Xie Qiao Wen and Nathan, C., 1997, Nitric oxide and macrophage function, *Annu. Rev. Immunol.*, **15**, 323–350

Maizels, R.M., Sartono, E., Kurniawan, A., Partono, F., Selkirk, M.E. and Yazdanbakhsh, M., 1995, T-cell activation and the balance of antibody isotypes in human lymphatic filariasis, *Parasitol. Today*, **11**, 50–56

Mansfield, J.M., 1995, Immunobiology of trypanosomiasis: a revisionist view, in Boothroyd, J.C. and Komuniecki, R. (eds) *Molecular Approaches to Parasitology*, New York: Wiley, pp. 477–496

Mauel, J., 1996, Intracellular survival of protozoan parasites with special reference to *Leishmania* spp., *Toxoplasma gondii* and *Trypanosoma cruzi*, *Adv. Parasitol.*, **38**, 1–51

Miles, M.A., 1998, New World trypanosomes, in Cox, F.E.G., Kreier, J.P. and Wakelin, D. (eds) *Topley and Wilson's Microbiology and Microbial Infections*, 9th edn, Vol. 5, *Parasitology*, London: Edward Arnold, pp. 283–302

Modabber, F., 1995, Vaccines against leishmaniasis, *Ann. Trop. Med. Parasitol.*, **89**, 83–88

Mosmann, T.R. and Sad, S., 1996, The expanding universe of T-cell subsets: T_H1, T_H2 and more, *Immunol. Today*, **17**, 138–146

Mountford, A.P. and Harrop, R., 1998, Vaccination against schistosomiasis: the case for lung stage antigens, *Parasitol. Today*, **14**, 109–114

Muller, R. and Wakelin, D., 1998, Lymphatic filariasis, in Cox, F.E.G., Kreier, J.P. and Wakelin, D. (eds) *Topley and Wilson's Microbiology and Microbial Infections*, 9th edn, Vol. 5, *Parasitology*, London: Edward Arnold, pp. 609–619

Nabors, G.S., 1997, Modulating ongoing T_H2-cell responses in experimental leishmaniasis, *Parasitol. Today*, **13**, 76–79

Nutman, T.B., 1995, Immune responses in lymphatic-dwelling filarial infections, in Boothroyd, J.C. and Komuniecki, R. (eds) *Molecular Approaches to Parasitology*, New York: Wiley, pp. 511–523

Pearce, E.J., 1995, The immunology of schistosomiasis, in Boothroyd, J.C. and Komuniecki, R. (eds) *Molecular Approaches to Parasitology*, New York: Wiley, pp. 497–510

Reed, S.G., 1998, Immunology of *Trypanosoma cruzi* infections, in Liew, F.Y. and Cox, F.E.G. (eds) *Immunology of Intracellular Parasitism, Chemical Immunology*, **70**, Basel: Karger, pp. 124–143

Reeder, J.C. and Brown, G.V., 1996, Antigenic variation and immune evasion in *Plasmodium falciparum* malaria, *Immunol. Cell Biol.*, **74**, 546–554

Riffkin, M., Seow, H.-F., Jackson, D., Brown, L. and Wood, P., 1996, Defence against the immune barrage: helminth survival strategies, *Immunol. Cell Biol.*, **74**, 564–574

Romagnani, S., 1997, Understanding the role of T_H1 and T_H2 cells in infection, *Trends Microbiol.*, **4**, 470–473

Seed, J.R., 1998, African trypanosomes, in Cox, F.E.G., Kreier, J.P. and Wakelin, D. (eds) *Topley and Wilson's Microbiology and Microbial Infections*, 9th edn, Vol. 5, *Parasitology*, London: Edward Arnold, pp. 267–282

Smith, N.C., Fell, A. and Good, M.F., 1998, Immunology of intracellular asexual blood stages of *Plasmodium*, in Liew, F.Y. and Cox, F.E.G. (eds) *Immunology of Intracellular Parasitism, Chemical Immunology*, **70**, Basel: Karger, pp. 144–161

Sternberg, J.M., 1998, Immunobiology of African try-panosomiasis, in Liew, F.Y. and Cox, F.E.G. (eds) *Immunology of Intracellular Parasitism, Chemical Immunology*, **70**, Basel: Karger, pp. 186–199

Targett, G.A.T., 1995, Malaria-advances in vaccines, *Curr. Opin. Infect. Dis.*, **8**, 322–327

Wakelin, D. 1996, *Immunity to Parasitic Infections: How Parasitic Infections are Controlled*, 2nd edn, Cambridge: Cambridge University Press

Warren, K.S. (ed.), 1993, *Immunology and Molecular Biology of Parasitic Infections*, Oxford: Blackwell Scientific Publications

Whitworth, J., 1998, Onchocerciasis, in Cox, F.E.G., Kreier, J.P. and Wakelin, D. (eds) *Topley and Wilson's Microbiology and Microbial Infections*, 9th edn, Vol. 5, *Parasitology*, London: Edward Arnold, pp. 621–633

Wynn, T.A., Cheever, A.W., Janovic, D., Poindexter, R.W., Caspar, P., Lewis, F.A. and Sher, A., 1995, An IL-12-based vaccination method for preventing fibrosis induced by schistosome infection, *Nature*, **376**, 594–596

5 Fungi

5.1 Classification of fungi

All fungi are eukaryotic heterotrophs, currently classified in the kingdoms Chromista, Fungi and Protozoa (Hawksworth *et al.*, 1995). As fungi lack chlorophyll they are unable to photosynthesize and require an external source of energy-containing carbon compounds in order to grow and reproduce. Fungi are thus either saprobic, deriving nutrients from dead organic matter, or parasitic, when they live on or within other living organisms, obtaining their food from and usually recognizably harming those organisms. An infection of a human or an animal caused by a fungus is termed a mycosis (plural mycoses). The aetiological agent is referred to as a mycopathogen. Most of the mycopathogens of human beings are also capable of living saprobically which, in the majority, constitutes the main non-parasitic phase of growth. In the saprobic phase, a mycopathogen may grow independently, be associated with a potential host as a commensal, or be regarded as a parasite but living, in fact, saprobically. Some pathogenic dermatophytes, such as *Epidermophyton* and *Trichophyton* species, appear to exist essentially as saprobes. They can be isolated from soil and the bodies of infected people and grown on nutrient media in the laboratory. On the human body, such dermatophytes grow saprobically on skin, hair and nails although they behave as pathogens, often being harmful to the human host. On the other hand, where no saprobic phase is known to occur in the life cycle, a mycopathogen may behave as an obligate parasite. Through careful and persistent experimentation, however, a method for culturing such organisms apart from the host on a nutrient medium (*in vitro*) is usually found, although none exists at present for *Loboa loboi*, the causal agent of cutaneous lobomycosis, and *Rhinosporidium seeberi*, responsible for nasal infections (Kwon-Chung, 1994). In *Pneumocystis carinii*, an organism responsible for the development of pneumonia, especially in patients with AIDS (acquired immune deficiency syndrome), no free-living form is known (Stringer and Walzer, 1996) and the organism appears to be restricted to growth in the living tissue of the lungs and viscera of humans and other mammals. Continuous *in vitro* growth of the strain of *P. carinii* which infects humans has not been achieved to date (Cailliez *et al.*, 1996) and it is consequently more difficult to study the growth characteristics of *P. carinii* in comparison with those fungi which can be readily cultured on nutrient media.

The soil constitutes a major reservoir of fungi pathogenic to humans and animals (Ajello, 1956). In the soil the fungus decays organic matter derived from the dead bodies of animals and plants and may grow and sporulate strongly. Mycopathogenic species of *Aspergillus* and members of the Mucorales (e.g. *Absidia*, *Mucor*, *Rhizopus*, see Figure 5.3) can usually be isolated from samples of topsoil and compost. Such fungi are essentially saprobic, acting as opportunistic (adventitious) mycopathogens, mainly infecting those who are already seriously ill and immunocompromised, or perhaps entering and infecting the bodies of otherwise healthy people through wounds. Some potential mycopathogens may also live saprobically as commensal organisms on the skin and mucocutaneous surfaces where they appear to constitute part of the normal microflora of the human body and cause no detectable damage. For example, species of *Aspergillus* may be isolated from the external auditory meatus and alveoli, and *Candida* from the skin of the hands and mucocutaneous surfaces of apparently healthy individuals.

Fungal classification (taxonomy) is complex and no single taxonomic system is universally accepted because the characters used to identify fungi and define taxa may be interpreted differently by different taxonomists. Thus judgements concerning the naming (nomenclature) and taxonomic position of individual fungi are, to some extent, subjective. Furthermore, ongoing discoveries relating to the structure, life cycle, genetic, physiological, biochemical and immunological characters of fungi influence taxonomists who determine and decide how a fungus should be named and where particular species should be placed within a taxonomic system. New information may stimulate both nomenclatural and taxonomic revision. *Pneumocystis carinii*, for example, long regarded as a member of the Protozoa is, on the basis of recent rRNA (ribosomal) sequencing information, currently considered to be a member of the Fungi (see the reviews of Cailliez *et al.*, 1996; Stringer and Walzer, 1996). The systematic position of *P. carinii* within the Fungi, however, is not clear. Current opinion favours placing *P. carinii* in the Ascomycota (Table 5.1) although it has previously been suggested that the organism may have an affinity with the Basidiomycota and the Zygomycota. Although only one species of *P. carinii* has been described, several variants are known to be associated with specific hosts, such as *P. carinii* sp. f. (special form)

Table 5.1 Taxonomic grouping of selected species of fungi recorded as pathogens of human beings (based on Hawksworth *et al.*, 1995)

KINGDOM CHROMISTA

PHYLUM HYPHOCHYTRIOMYCOTA
RHINOSPORIDIUM seeberi

KINGDOM FUNGI

PHYLUM ASCOMYCOTA
*AJELLOMYCES dermatitidis, A. capsulata; ALTERNARIA alternata, A. tenuis; ASPERGILLUS flavus, A. fumigatus, A. glaucus, A. granulosus, A. nidulans, A. niger, A. terreus; BIPOLARIS spicifera; BLASTOMYCES dermatitidis; CANDIDA albicans, C. glabrata, C. guillermondii, C. krusei, C. lusitaniae, C. parapsilosis, C. rugosa, C. tropicalis; CLADOSPORIUM carrionii, C. trichoides, C. werneckii; CURVULARIA lunata; DRECHSLERA hawaiiensii, D. rostrata; EXSEROHILUM longirostratum; FUSARIUM moniliforme, F. proliferatum, F. solani; GEOTRICHUM candidum, G. capitatum, G. clavatum; HISTOPLASMA capsulatum; MICROSPORUM audouinii, M. canis, M. ferrugineum, M. gypseum, M. langeroni, M. nanum, M. rivalieri; ONYCHOCOLA canadensis; PAECILOMYCES lilacinus, P. variotii; PENICILLIUM chrysogenum, P. decumbens, P. marneffei; PHIALOPHORA americana, P. parasitica, P. pedrosoi, P. repens, P. verrucosa; PICHIA anomala, P. fabianii, P. polymorpha; *PIEDRAIA hortae; PNEUMOCYSTIS carinii; *PSEUDALLESCHERIA boydii; *SACCHAROMYCES cerevisiae; SCEDOSPORIUM inflatum; SCOPULARIOPSIS brevicaulis; SPOROTHRIX schenckii; TRICHODERMA koningii, T. longibrachiatum; T. viride; TRICHOPHYTON concentricum, T. mentagrophytes, T. rubrum, T. schoenleinii, T. tonsurans, T. violaceum

PHYLUM BASIDIOMYCOTA
*COPRINUS cinereus; CRYPTOCOCCUS neoformans; *FILOBASIDIELLA neoformans; *SCHIZOPHYLLUM commune; *USTILAGO sp.

PHYLUM ZYGOMYCOTA
*ABSIDIA corymbifera; *APOPHYSOMYCES elegans; *BASIDIOBOLUS haptosporus, B. meristosporus, B. ranarum; *COKEROMYCES recurvatus; *CONIDIOBOLUS coronatus, C. incongruus; *CUNNINGHAMELLA berthollettiae; *MORTIERELLA wolfii; *MUCOR circinelloides, M. indicus, M. racemosus; *RHIZOMUCOR pusillus; *RHIZOPUS arrhizus, R. microsporus, R. oligosporus, R. rhizopodiformis, R. stolonifer; SAKSENAEA vasiformis; *SYNCEPHALASTRUM racemosum

MITOSPORIC FUNGI
ACREMONIUM alabamensis; AUREOBASIDIUM pullulans; COCCIDIODES immitis; EPIDERMOPHYTON floccosum; EXOPHIALA dermatitidis, E. jeanselmei; MADURELLA grisea, M. mycetomatis; MALASSEZIA furfur, M. pachydermatitis; PARACOCCIDIODES brasiliensis; PHAEOANNELLOMYCES werneckii; RHODOTORULA minuta, R. rubra; SPOROBOLOMYCES roseus, S. salmonicolor; TRICHOSPORON asahii, T. asteroides, T. beigelii, T. inkin, T. mucoides, T. ovoides

* teleomorph (sexual), the remainder in Ascomycota, Basidiomycota and Zygomycota are anamorphic (asexual) with known teleomorphic affinities.
Sporobolomyces appears to have an affinity with Basidiomycota.
No zygospores have been found in *Saksenaea*.

hominis – human, *P. carinii* sp. f. *carinii* – rat, *P. carinii* sp. f. *muris* – mouse, and so on (Cailliez *et al.*, 1996). Whether more than one species is involved in this complex remains to be determined.

Most of the mycopathogenic fungi are referred to the kingdom of Fungi. Table 5.1 provides a guide to the classification of selected mycopathogens of humans and is not intended to be exhaustive. Members of the phylum Ascomycota, in which the majority of known mycopathogens of humans are either included or are associated, are characterized by the production of meiospores, the products of meiosis, within a sporangium (spore-containing structure) termed an ascus. Typically, although not invariably, a mature ascus contains eight ascospores; that of the yeast *Saccharomyces cerevisiae* normally contains four (Figure 5.1). With the exception of *Ajellomyces*, *Piedraia*, *Pseudallescheria* and *Saccharomyces*, however, the genera of Ascomycota in Table 5.1 are anamorphs (asexual state), their teleomorphs (sexual state) being referred to different genera which are known to produce ascospores.

Basidiomycota are characterized by the production of meiospores on an element termed the basidium. Usually four basidiospores are produced externally per basidium, each poised at the apex of a delicate projection (sterigma) prior to liberation into the atmosphere (Figure 5.1). Although few of the Basidiomycota appear to be responsible for the development of mycotic infections, it is worth noting that the toadstools are included in this phylum and that the spores of many of these are known to be potentially allergenic (see review by Horner *et al.*, 1995). In the autumn especially, in woodlands and grasslands of the United Kingdom, throughout Europe and elsewhere in the world, many species of toadstool sporulate profusely liberating millions of basidiospores into the atmosphere. Susceptible individuals may develop respiratory problems through the inhalation of airborne basidiospores.

Zygomycota are characterized by the fusion of the gametangia resulting in the production of a zygosporangium which contains a single resting zygospore (Figure 5.1). The zygosporangium is frequently thick-walled and is thought usually to be associated with meiosis during development or on germination.

Mitosporic fungi (= Deuteromycotina = Fungi Imperfecti) lack meiospores but may produce asexual spores or remain sterile. Some mitosporic fungi (anamorphic) can be related to meiosporic (teleomorphic) Ascomycota or Basidiomycota. For example, *Cryptococcus neoformans* is the anamorph of *Filobasidiella neoformans* (Basidiomycota) the teleomorph.

Figure 5.1
Morphology of fungi.
Diagrammatic and not to scale.
(a) Radial growth of mycelium in a Petri dish; (b) aerial sporulation; (c) non-septate hypha;
(d) septate hypha; (e) clamp connexion; (f) *Apophysomyces* asexual sporangia; (g)
Schizophyllum ventral surface of basidiocarp with split gills; (h) *Cryptococcus neoformans*
encapsulated yeast cells; (i) *Sporobolomyces* with a ballistospore; (j) Y-phase *Cokeromyces*
with buds (blastospores); (k) *Saccharomyces* budding; (l) zygosporangium; (m) tetrasporic
basidium; (n) tetrasporic ascus, e.g. *Saccharomyces*; (o) arthrospores; (p) chlamydospores;
(q) *Conidiobolus* with ballistospore; (r) *Conidiobolus* appendaged resting spore;
(s) *Basidiobolus* with ballistospore; (t) *Basidiobolus* zygosporangium; (u) *Aspergillus*
conidial head; (v) *Aspergillus flavus* sclerotium; (w) *Penicillium* conidial head.

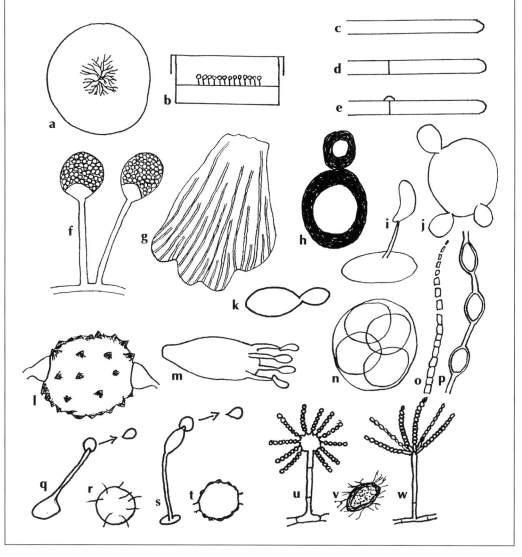

Hyphochytriomycota (kingdom Chromista) possess a zoospore with a single anterior flagellum.

5.1.1 *Further characteristics of fungi*

The fungal thallus may be unicellular as in many yeasts or filamentous. Yeast is a general term referring to unicellular fungi which produce buds (blastospores) or undergo fission. Different genera of yeasts may be unrelated, for example *Saccharomyces cerevisiae*, the brewer's or baker's yeast (Ascomycota); *Cryptococcus neoformans* (Figure 5.1), an encapsulated yeast (Basidiomycota), mirror image yeast and the mitosporic *Sporobolomyces roseus* (Figure 5.1). Some filamentous fungi may also produce a yeast phase (Y-phase), *Cokeromyces recurvatus*, for example (Figure 5.1), develops multibudding yeast elements when grown on a yeast–peptone medium (Jeffries and Young, 1983).

An individual element of the thallus of a filamentous fungus is termed a hypha. Sporangiospores of fast-growing Zygomycota such as species of *Absidia* (Figure 5.3), *Mucor* (Figure 5.3) or *Rhizopus* (Figure 5.3) plated onto nutrient media in 9 cm Petri dishes incubated at 25°C may develop germ tubes within a few hours which branch forming a hyphal mass or mycelium (Figure 5.1). The mycelium (M-phase) can cover the surface of plates inoculated in the centre within 24 h and aerial sporulation may also occur profusely after 24 to 48 h (Figure 5.1). Hyphae in these genera are broad and do not normally develop cross-walls (septa) except where reproductive structures are formed or when they are damaged (Figure 5.1). Hyphae in members of the Ascomycota, Basidiomycota and Mitosporic fungi are septate (Figure 5.1). Fungi having both a Y-phase and an M-phase or two recognizably distinct asexual phases in the life cycle are said to be dimorphic or biphasic (Figure 5.2).

The hyphal wall in pathogenic mycelial members of the kingdom Fungi contains a high proportion of chitin, and that of the yeasts mannan-glucan (e.g. *Cryptococcus*, *Saccharomyces*) or mannan-chitin (e.g. *Sporobolomyces*), together with other components which may act as antigens or virulence factors in the pathogenic stage of these fungi (San-Blas, 1982). For example, elements of *Candida albicans* adhere firmly to cells of the buccal cavity, cervix and many other types of surface making them difficult to dislodge and it is thought that wall chemistry could have a significant role in the process of adhesion (Kennedy *et al.*, 1988; Vartivarian, 1992). Blastospores of the pathogenic yeast *Cryptococcus neoformans* have a thick polysaccharide capsule which enables the cells to resist phagocytosis (Murphy, 1991). Hyphae in some Basidiomycota, such as *Schizophyllum commune*, a causal agent of basidiomycosis, also possess clamp connexions (Figure 5.1) which are found over septa and can be a useful aid in the identification of this infection.

Hyphae grow apically and penetrate both solid and liquid substrates, including human tissues. Extracellular enzymes, such as lipases and proteases which are secreted, digest the substrate and the soluble products are absorbed over the surface area, which is high in relation to the volume enabling further, often rapid, growth to occur. Extracellular digestion of organic materials is responsible for their decay and may be accompanied by musty or mouldy odours, for example in damp housing. The spores of fungi which may sporulate profusely under such conditions, such as species of *Aspergillus* and *Penicillium*, often referred to as moulds, may be responsible for the development of respiratory allergies. Extracellular enzyme activity also contributes to pathogenic virulence and may be of importance in those infections where necrosis of tissue occurs, for example protease secretion in zygomycoses. Dermatophytes, such as *Trichophyton* species and the yeast *Candida albicans*, secrete keratinases that enable penetration and colonization of the stratum corneum to occur (Wagner and Sohnle, 1995). Extracellular elastase which digests elastin in the epithelium of the lung, produced by hyphae of *Aspergillus fumigatus*, probably enables this pathogen to establish pulmonary infections (Tomee *et al.*, 1994). Similarly, the extracellular proteases of *Candida albicans* and *Coccidiodes immitis* may enhance their virulence (Murphy, 1991). A virulence factor of the conidiospores of *A. fumigatus* is the rapid diffusibility from the spore of a substance which inhibits the chemotactic movement and phagocytic ability of macrophages. The hyphae also produce gliotoxin, an antibiotic also known to depress macrophage function (Seaton and Robertson, 1989). Secondary metabolites (formed after the primary phase of growth in length) of some filamentous fungi, such as *Aspergillus*, *Fusarium* and *Penicillium* species, are also known to be poisonous (mycotoxins) and it is possible that such compounds could augment the process of infection by a mycopathogen.

The mycelium may also produce distinctive vegetative structures. Arthrospores (= arthroconidiospores, appearing jointed) may develop when the elements of a septate hypha separate into numerous propagules, for example in *Coccidiodes immitis*, *Geotrichum candidum*, *Onychocola canadensis*, and *Trichosporon beigelii* (Figure 5.1). In the filamentous pathogenic yeast *Candida albicans*, the hyphal elements which can be loosely aggregated may separate, akin to arthrospores, and this phase is referred to as a pseudomycelium (Figure 5.2). Perennating chlamydospores (Figure 5.1), which arise within hyphal elements by the condensation of areas of cytoplasm becoming surrounded by a spore wall that is often but not invariably thickened, may develop both terminally and in an intercalary position in the mycelium, for example in *C. albicans*, *Fusarium solani*, *Mortierella wolfii*, and *Mucor racemosus*. Chlamydospores are known to develop in the tissues of patients with cutaneous and pulmonary zygomycosis (Chandler *et al.*, 1985).

Aggregation of hyphae into discrete, dense rind-bound, tough perennating sclerotia (Figure 5.1) which lodge in the tissues, for example in *Aspergillus flavus*, may enhance pathogenicity through resistance to the penetration of antifungal antibiotics (Frank *et al.*, 1988).

Individual fungi may grow over a wide range of temperature. For those working with living fungi in laboratories it is prudent to assume that any fungus capable of growing at body temperature (37°C) could be potentially pathogenic. Dermatophytes, nevertheless, also survive well at the lower temperatures associated with the external surface of the human body. Fungi are often grown in science laboratories for reasons other than those associated with medicine and it is important for those experimenting with them to be aware that these organisms could be a potential source of health problems. For example, the author has experimented with *Cokeromyces recurvatus* (Figure 5.3) for over 30 years as it is very conveniently grown in the laboratory at 25°C on nutrient media. It is a Y-phase/M-phase fungus used as a standard host to infect with mycoparasitic fungi such as species of *Piptocephalis* (see Jeffries and Young, 1994). Although this organism was not usually regarded as a pathogen of humans, there have been reports since the late 1970s of this species causing urinogenital problems (Kemna *et al.*, 1994). Similarly, species of *Conidiobolus* and *Basidiobolus* (Figure 5.1), cultured for experiments on spore discharge and hyphal growth, are causal agents of subcutaneous entomophthoromycosis. *Schizophyllum commune* (Figure 5.1), a bracket toadstool with split gills which produces basidiocarps (toadstools) very readily in culture, again used for growth, sporulation and genetic experiments, is known to be responsible for pulmonary and brain infections (Rihs *et al.*, 1996). Staff and patients in hospitals are also at risk from nosocomial (hospital-acquired) mycoses (Ahearn and Price, 1995; Sewell, 1995; see section 5.3.4).

Morphology of the asexual sporulation apparatus of mycopathogenic fungi may be distinctive enabling generic and often specific identifications to be made (Figures 5.2 and 5.3). Species of *Rhizopus* and *Absidia* develop stoloniferous hyphae which may rapidly cover a surface in every direction including the lids of Petri dishes. Where the stoloniferous hyphae touch down they are normally anchored by dark-coloured (*Rhizopus*), short rhizoidal hyphae. In *Rhizopus* the aerial sporangiophores (hyphae which bear sporangia) develop in small groups where the stoloniferous hyphae touch down, whereas in *Absidia* the sporangiophores develop along the aerial part of the stoloniferous hyphae. Conidiospores, asexual spores other than those developed within sporangia, develop on hyphae termed conidiophores. In Petri dish culture, the conidiospores of species of *Aspergillus* and *Penicillium* and the sporangiospores of *Rhizopus* are formed in great profusion under aerobic conditions. Great care has to be taken not to inhale the spores when handling such fungi as all species of *Aspergillus*, *Penicillium* and *Rhizopus* produce dry spores which are readily liberated into the atmosphere at maturity from the sporulation apparatus by the slightest air turbulence. In *Mucor*, stoloniferous hyphae are absent, the sporangiophores which may be branched or unbranched arise directly from the substratum, and the sporangiospores are either dry or embedded in slime at maturity according to species. The sporangial apparatus in *Mucor* and its allies (Mucorales) may be distinctive and diagnostic (Figure 5.3). The sporangia in Mucorales are frequently columellate, that is with a septum which is often characteristic in form, which separates the sporangium from the sporangiophore. The columella in the dehisced sporangium of *Rhizopus* frequently collapses into a characteristic inverted pudding bowl shape (Figure 5.3). Sporangia of *Mortierella* species (Figure 5.3) either lack a columella or possess a rudimentary one. *Saksenaea vasiformis* has a unique elongate vasiform multispored sporangium (Figure 5.3). The recurved pedicellate sporangioles (small sporangia) of *Cokeromyces recurvatus* (Figure 5.3) and the linear sporangioles of *Syncephalastrum racemosum* (Figure 5.3) each contain only a few sporangiospores. The usually distinctly spinose sporangiole of *Cunninghamella* species (Figure 5.3) contains a single sporangiospore. In *Cokeromyces*, *Cunninghamella* and *Syncephalastrum* the entire sporangiole is liberated at maturity (Young, 1969). Figures 5.1 to 5.3 outline the range of form of some mycopathogenic fungi.

Spore form can also be a useful character in diagnosis of the mycotic agent. The unicellular ovoid sporangiospores of *Rhizopus* appear striate, the septate macroconidia of *Fusarium* are lunate and sometimes also contain chlamydospores. In

Figure 5.2

Some dimorphic mycopathogens.

Diagrammatic and not to scale.

Blastomyces dermatitidis: (a) bud on a broad base, (b) conidial M-phase; *Candida albicans*: (c) Y-phase budding, (d) M-phase budding and a germinating blastospore; *Coccidioides immitis*: (e) spherule containing endospores, (f) arthrosporic M-phase; *Histoplasma capsulatum*: (g) Y-phase, (h) M-phase with microconidia and macroconidia; *Sporothrix schenckii*: (i) Y-phase, (j) conidial M-phase.

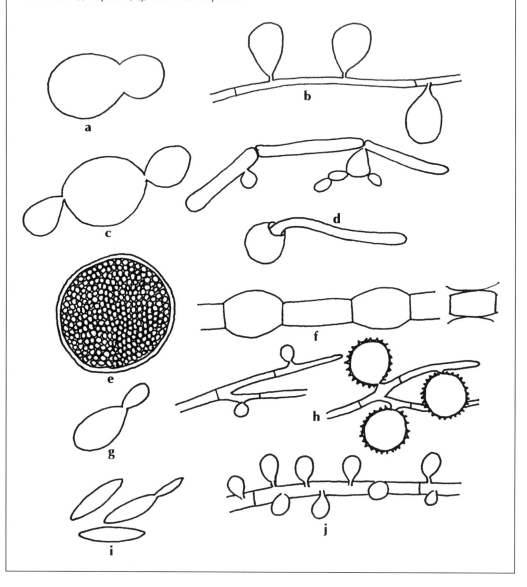

Figure 5.3

Zygomycosis: asexual apparatus of Mucorales.

Diagrammatic and not to scale.

(a) *Absidia*, sporangiophores arise from stoloniferous hyphae, sporangia multispored;

(b) *Mucor*, sporangiophores arise from hyphae in substratum, sporangia multispored;

(c) *Rhizopus*, sporangiophores arise from stoloniferous hyphae near dark-coloured rhizoidal hyphae, sporangia multispored, sporangiospores always dry; (d) *Saksenaea* with a vasiform multispored sporangium; (e) *Cunninghamella* with detachable one-spored sporangia;

(f) *Mortierella* with few-spored sporangia; (g) *Syncephalastrum* with detachable few-spored rod-like sporangia; (h) *Cokeromyces* with detachable few-spored spherical sporangia.

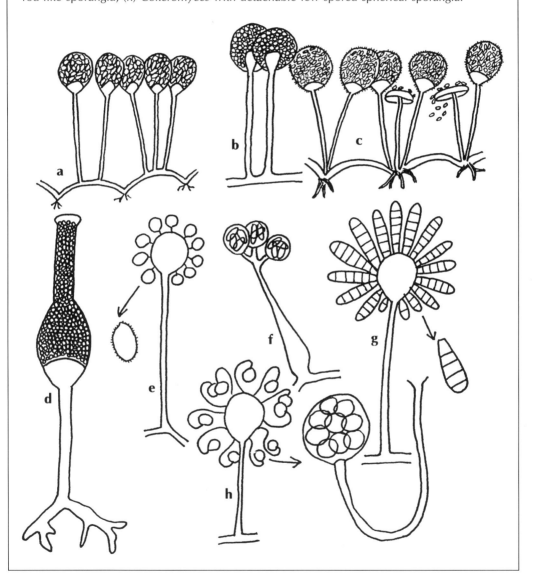

Alternaria the wall of the muriform (septa in more than one plane) obclavate conidiospore is pigmented brown (dematiaceous) and the conidiospores are either solitary or may adhere in short chains. Conidiospores, which arise singly in the keratinophilic *Microsporum* species, are large, thick-walled and often ornamented appearing roughened under the light microscope. Basidiospores of toadstools (Pegler and Young, 1971) and the ballistospore of *Sporobolomyces* (Figure 5.1) always have a hilar appendix, a minute projection of the spore attached to the sterigma before violent discharge from the basidium, a convex abaxial surface and an adaxial surface often with some degree of applanation (flattening). Knowledge of the form and structure of basidiospores is important to the physician in the diagnosis and treatment of cases of poisoning due to the ingestion of poisonous toadstools (mycetism).

Laboratory methods for the diagnosis of a range of mycoses include microscopical examination of clinical specimens obtained by biopsy, swabs and scrapings of infected areas of the body, sputum and body fluids, especially blood in cases of fungaemia, and growth of the suspected organism in culture where possible. Every organ and tissue in the human body appears to be vulnerable to fungal infection (Male, 1991). Various histological staining techniques have been devised to assist diagnosis of the mycotic agents. Non-microscopical techniques involve antigen and radioimmunoassays (Musial *et al.*, 1988; Kaufman, 1992).

5.2 Global significance of mycoses

In the first half of the twentieth century human mycoses were rare in comparison with other forms of infection. Since the 1950s, concomitant with advances in medicine involving the development and use of antibiotics, immunosuppressive drugs, steroid and contraceptive hormonal preparations, and organ transplantation, infections due to fungi have increased dramatically. Antibacterial antibiotic and chemotherapeutic treatments may also alter the normal ecological balance of the microflora of the body in favour of mycopathogens. It has been estimated that in up to 25 per cent of the population of the world, mycoses constitute the most frequently occurring infections (Male, 1991) and vast expenditure is now incurred annually on antifungal treatments. Populations in many countries are also ageing with many more people than formerly surviving into old age. Any decline in immun-ocompetence through ageing and malnutrition is likely to be accompanied by increased risk of fungal infection. The acceleration in AIDS since 1983 and the current resurgence of tuberculosis through multidrug resistance are often associated with several fungal infections which are difficult to treat in such patients and may persist. The ease with which people are transported around the world enables intercontinental barriers to sexually transmitted *Candida* infections and fungus-related illness due to AIDS to be readily broken. The illegal global use of drugs through intravenous injection in unsterile conditions can lead to fungaemia and other forms of mycosis and constitutes a cause for concern.

Some mycoses occur worldwide whilst others are more localized in distribution. Table 5.2 shows a range of mycoses afflicting human beings, their main causal agents and effects on the body. The descriptive terms are not consistent as, for example, basidiomycosis and zygomycosis (= mucormycosis = phycomycosis) refer to particular groups of fungi; alternariasis, aspergillosis and candidiasis refer to genera and dermatophytosis, onychomycosis and pneumomycosis apply to the infected part of the body. These terms and many others are, however, frequently used. Dermatophytosis involving cutaneous infection of the head, limbs and body occurs in populations throughout the world, although not necessarily with the same frequency in different populations (Binazzi *et al.*, 1983). The manifestations of aspergillosis, candidiasis, cryptococcosis, onychomycosis and zygomycosis are also known to occur in patients globally. With cryptococcosis there is a well-defined association between the incidence of disease and prior contact with the faeces of birds, especially pigeons and sometimes caged birds. Paracoccidiomycosis, on the other hand, is endemic in parts of Latin America and the disease appears more frequently in males than females (48:1) in Colombia, possibly due to hormonal differences (Restrepo *et al.*, 1984). Apparently, delay or reduction in the rate of transformation of the M- to Y-phase in the lungs due to oestrogen could be a contributory factor to the marked resistance of females to this disease. Coccidiomycosis is endemic in arid parts of the south-western United States, Mexico and South America, and may also occur in other areas of the globe (Stevens, 1995). The incidence of cocci-diomycosis, however, is higher in pregnant individuals than in the general population. Blastomycosis caused by *Blastomyces dermatitidis* is endemic in the south-eastern and mid-western areas of the United States (Harrell and Curtis,

Table 5.2 Selected mycoses, principal aetiological genera and main infection sites (compiled from and based on various sources including English, 1980; Male, 1991; Kwon-Chung, 1994)

Mycosis	Genus	Main infection site
Alternariasis	*Alternaria*	Dermal granuloma, meninges
Aspergillosis	*Aspergillus*	Lung, vascular system, CNS, systemic
Basidiomycosis	*Schizophyllum*	Nasal sinus, brain, lung, nail
Blastomycosis	*Blastomyces*	Lung, skin, bone, eye, brain, systemic
Candidiasis	*Candida*	Mucous membranes, fungaemia, systemic
Chromomycosis	*Phialophora*	Skin, septic arthritis, systemic
Coccidiomycosis	*Coccidiodes*	Lung, bone, joints, systemic
Cryptococcosis	*Cryptococcus*	Lung, brain, systemic
Dermatophytosis	*Epidermophyton*	Cutaneous, keratinophilic
	Microsporum	Stratum corneum, hair shaft, nail
	Trichophyton	Stratum corneum, hair shaft, nail
Entomophthoromycosis	*Basidiobolus*	Subcutaneous: palate, limbs, trunk, gut
	Conidiobolus	Subcutaneous: rhinofacial
Fusariosis	*Fusarium*	Subcutaneous: leg; fungaemia, systemic
Geotrichosis	*Geotrichum*	Lung and brain abscesses, septicaemia
Histoplasmosis	*Histoplasma*	Lung, systemic
Hyalohyphomycosis	*Fusarium*	Lung, systemic
	Penicillium	Liver, subcutaneous abscess, systemic
Keratomycosis	*Aspergillus*	Corneal ulcers, microabscesses
	Curvularia	Corneal ulcers, microabscesses
	Fusarium	Corneal ulcers, microabscesses
Maduramycosis	*Madurella*	Subcutaneous: mycetoma of limbs
	Pseudallescheria	Subcutaneous: limbs; lung, systemic
Onychomycosis	*Candida*	Tissue of nail folds
	Onychocola	Nail, skin
	Trichophyton	Keratin of damaged nails
Otomycosis	*Aspergillus*	External auditory meatus
Paracoccidiomycosis	*Paracoccidioides*	Lungs, skin, systemic
Phaeohyphomycosis	*Aureobasidium*	Brain abscess
	Bipolaris	Skin, paranasal sinus
Pityriasis	*Malassezia*	Cutaneous: skin
Pneumomycosis	*Pneumocystis*	Lungs, especially in AIDS, systemic
Rhinosporidiosis	*Rhinosporidium*	Nasal polyps, brain
Sporotrichosis	*Sporothrix*	Subcutaneous: limbs, lymphatic system
Torulopsidosis	*Pichia*	Fungaemia (septicaemia), prostatitis
	Rhodotorula	Fungaemia
	Saccharomyces	Fungaemia
	Sporobolomyces	Skin, madura foot, fungaemia
Trichosporonosis	*Trichosporon*	Hair, brain, systemic
Ustilagomycosis	*Ustilago*	Meninges
Zygomycosis	*Absidia*	Wounds, vascular, rhinocerebral, systemic
	Apophysomyces	Osteomyelitis, vascular, systemic
	Cokeromyces	Cervix, bladder
	Cunninghamella	Lungs, systemic
	Mortierella	Rhinocerebral
	Mucor	Skin, rhinocerebral
	Rhizopus	Wounds, rhinocerebral, lung, bone
	Saksenaea	Wounds, subcutaneous, brain, systemic
	Syncephalastrum	Skin, rhinocerebral

1959). Histoplasmosis due to *Histoplasma capsulatum* (North American histoplasmosis) is endemic in central areas of the USA, particularly the Mississippi and Ohio river valleys, parts of Latin America, Africa, Asia and Europe, whilst that caused by *H. duboisii* (African histoplasmosis) is endemic in Africa and Madagascar (Manfredi *et al.*, 1994). The geographical areas in which blastomycosis and North American histoplasmosis occur overlap (Wheat, 1995). The causal agents of entomophthoromycosis although occurring widely, for instance in South America and Australia, and maduramycosis in Africa, India and South America, tend to thrive as mycopathogens in the tropical areas of those continents (Mahe *et al.*, 1996).

Although healthy people are probably exposed to propagules of potentially pathenogenic fungi daily, they tend to remain uninfected. The skin, with its competing community of microorganisms, exposure to irradiation in sunlight, with lower temperature and moisture relations than the interior of the body, presents a formidable natural barrier to infection by mycopathogens. When an apparently healthy person acquires a fungal infection, due perhaps to exposure to an unusually high inoculum of infective units which are inhaled, or by accidental inoculation through the skin, the disease is regarded as a primary mycosis. For example, infection of healthy lung tissue (Ahmad *et al.*, 1984; Andersen *et al.*, 1985) or the larynx (Kheir *et al.*, 1983) by *Aspergillus* species (Figure 5.1) may cause primary pulmonary aspergillosis and primary laryngeal aspergillosis. Primary pulmonary zygomycosis (Ferrinho, 1985) and wound zygomycosis (Vainrub *et al.,* 1988) are also known. Species of *Fusarium*, normally considered to be root-infecting pathogens, may be responsible for abscess formation and ulceration of the feet of otherwise healthy patients (Willemsen *et al.*, 1986; Leu *et al.*, 1995). The accidental inoculation or inhalation of the infective agents of blastomycosis, coccidiomycosis and histoplasmosis by employees handling the organisms in laboratories has resulted in primary infections (Howard, 1984). It is important for those whose work involves the growth of mycopathogens in culture to recognize that they could be exposed to massive dosages of inocula which are likely to far exceed the concentrations of infective propagules found in a natural habitat such as humified soil. Dermatophytoses due to the keratinophilous dermatophytes are probably mainly primary in nature. Traumatic injury to the skin sustained through vehicle accidents may result, for example, in primary zygomycosis or penetration by wood splinters and other plant materials in sporotrichosis.

5.2.1 *Predisposing factors to mycoses*

Secondary mycoses, however, may develop when the physiological state and health of the host is already compromised and the weakened body cannot resist sufficiently to overcome the infection. Physical, chemical and biological conditions which enhance the susceptibility of the body to fungal infection and may influence the course of disease are referred to as predisposing factors. At risk from fungal infections, particularly aspergillosis, candidiasis and cryptococcosis, are those with serious pre-existing illnesses such as AIDS and tuberculosis. Penicilliosis, due to *Penicillium marneffei*, is endemic in Hong Kong and Thailand where it is regarded as an AIDS-defining illness (Fenelon, 1997). Patients with insulin-dependent hyperglycaemia may be affected by zygomycosis and candidiasis. Other endocrine deficiencies, such as hypothyroidism, or an abnormal hormonal balance, may increase susceptibility of the body to candidiasis. Malignant disorders such as tumorous cancers, Hodgkin's disease, leukaemia, other haematological problems, immunological deficiencies and chronic granulomatous disease put patients at risk from systemic aspergillosis and candidiasis. Exocrine-related cystic fibrosis may predispose patients to pulmonary aspergillosis (Arruda *et al.*, 1995). The genetic constitution of the individual may also be related to susceptibility to fungal infection. Inability of the polymorphonuclear leucocytes to produce peroxidases which catalyse reactions involving the production of antifungal hydrogen peroxide and other fungitoxic materials is associated with X-linked chronic granulomatous disease in males.

Use of antibacterial antibiotics and antibacterial chemotherapeutic drugs, especially when the treatment is extensive and prolonged, may also alter the balance of the normal microflora of the body allowing fungi to gain the ascendancy, possibly stimulating the tendency toward pathogenicity. In dual bacterial/fungal infections, antibacterial treatment given either alone or until the fungal infection is also diagnosed could exacerbate the mycosis. Patients with cancer treated with antimitotic drugs or subjected to X-irradiation may also be susceptible to aspergillosis and candidiasis. The requirement for treatment with immunosuppressive agents such as corticosteroids in organ and tissue transplant surgery (e.g. liver, renal, heart, lung, bone marrow) may also expose the patients to the infective agents of aspergillosis, cryptococcosis and zygomycosis. These mycoses are severe and can be lethal.

Surgical procedures themselves may expose patients to mycotic infections. Indwelling catheters which allow movement of fluid, for instance from the bladder or peritoneum, or intravascular fluids, may be associated with fungaemia due to *Candida* and other yeasts. Surgically implanted plastic venous catheters which enable the patient to receive nutrients, antibiotic and chemotherapeutic fluids, and blood products may remain in place for over 9 months. It seems, however, that fungaemia due to *Rhodotorula*, other yeasts (Kiehn *et al.*, 1992; Goldani *et al.*, 1995), *Fusarium oxysporum* (Raad and Hachem, 1995) and *Paecilomyces lilacinus* (Fenelon, 1997), sometimes occurs with intravenous catheter usage. The application of wound dressings to the skin after surgery or burns, through providing a combination of warmth, moisture and pressure or tension which may macerate the underlying wound tissue, can also provide a microenvironment favourable to growth and infection by, for example, *Rhizopus* and other members of the Mucorales.

Physical, physiological and chemical changes associated with the skin and mucous membranes may lead to increased susceptibility to mycotic infections. Persistent abrasion of the epithelium of the buccal cavity through poorly fitting dentures, which can occur in elderly people where the gums recede during ageing, may predispose the individual to thrush, a manifestation of candidiasis. Cream-coloured colonies of the yeast adhere firmly to the buccal cavity, tongue and throat making feeding painful and difficult. In the elderly, immunocompetence usually declines and in neonates, time is required for the immune system to develop fully. Both groups of individuals may be afflicted by oral and anal candidiasis.

Vaginal candidiasis can affect women when the pH rises and *Lactobacillus acidophilus* is replaced by *Candida* species. During pregnancy, the development of vaginal thrush appears related to oestrogen activity. An increase in concentration of glycogen and change in pH due to the hormone improve adhesion of the fungus to the vaginal epithelium. The flow of leucocytes to the vagina is also reduced and susceptibility to infection increased (Murphy, 1991). Prolonged exposure of the hands to water through washing dishes and clothing, for example, may remove protective long-chain fatty acids from the skin, and a combination of warmth and moisture in skin folds of the body may predispose the individual to onychomycosis and cutaneous candidiasis. Excessive perspiration (hyperhidrosis), overactive sebaceous glands (seborrhoea) and physical damage (trauma) to the skin may all predispose people to fungal infections.

Persistent exposure to a potential source of infection may result in fungal allergies, chronic lung infections and systemic mycoses. A mycosis could develop during the course of an occupation which involves exposure to potentially pathogenic fungi. *Aspergillus fumigatus* and other microorganisms have been implicated in respiratory illness in farmers (farmer's lung disease), mushroom growers, grain millers and woodworkers in saw mills (Lacey, 1991). Grain handlers, for example, inhaling spores and fragments of mycelium or physically contacting contaminated material may also be exposed to mycotoxins, secondary metabolites known to be cytotoxic in high dilution, produced by fungi such as *Aspergillus*, *Fusarium* and *Penicillium* associated with plants and the soil. Some mycotoxins are known to reduce immunocompetence in farm and experimental animals and exposure to these poisons should, if possible, be avoided. Malnutrition also reduces immunocompetence and increases susceptibility to infection. In those areas of the world where communities may have to rely on the consumption of mouldy grain, perhaps conserving the best grain for crop planting, such individuals may be exposed to debilitating or lethal mycotoxicoses in addition to mycotic infections. Exposure to mycoses may also be self-induced where people are addicted to drugs. Cirrhosis of the liver due to alcoholism, smoking marijuana and the intravenous injection of heroin with dirty hypodermic syringes can also predispose individuals to aspergillosis, candidiasis and zygomycosis. Cirrhosis reduces immunocompetence. Inhalation of tobacco smoke containing the conidiospores of potentially infective aspergilli and other fungi increases the risk of hypersensitivity pneumonitis and bronchopulmonary infections. Intravascular inoculation of unsterile drugs, such as heroin, may also inject a dose of fungal inoculum sufficient to initiate tissue infection or fungaemia.

5.2.2 *Immunity to mycoses*

Reviews of the mechanisms of resistance of humans to fungal pathogens have been published (e.g. Murphy, 1986, 1991; Cassadevall, 1995; Wagner and Sohnle, 1995). Mechanisms of resistence are complex and only a brief introduction is provided here. Healthy individuals display immunity to fungal infections through two main lines of defence, the physicochemical barrier of intact skin and mucocutaneous areas, and the immune system.

Continuous shedding of the stratum corneum may also remove superficial fungal pathogens. Inflammation due to secretion of soluble factors, such as cytokines by microvascular endothelial cells, tends to enhance proliferation of the epidermis which increases the rate of sloughing. Sebum, sphingosines and lipids in hair are fungistatic (i.e. stopping growth but not killing). The iron-binding fungistatic protein unsaturated transferrin may restrict growth of dermatoyphytes to the keratinized layer by competition for iron in the dermis. The skin has been described as an immune surveillance unit (Wagner and Sohnle, 1995). Major antigens in the fungal wall of dermatophytes are carbohydrates, glycopeptides and peptides, which may stimulate protective cutaneous immunological responses via epidermal Langerhans cells, dermal dendritic cells, keratinocytes and T lymphocytes. Epidermal Langerhans cells, for example, phagocytose and react with antigens, presenting them for fungitoxic T-lymphocyte activation.

The natural cellular defence of the body against mycopathogens also involves polymorphonuclear leucocytes and cytokine-activated macrophages, which ingest or attach to fungal elements and may kill them intracellularly through phagocytosis and extracellularly by oxidative reactions, for instance the myeloperoxidase–hydrogen peroxide route, or by oxygen-independent reactions involving, for example, hydrolytic enzymes (Murphy, 1986). The ability of alveolar macrophages to kill varies with the type of pathogen, which highlights the complexity of the defence mechanisms. Conidiospores of *Aspergillus* species are normally prevented from infecting the lung; cells of *Cryptococcus neoformans* although usually prevented from infecting vary in susceptibility according to strain, whilst infective propagules of *Coccidiodes immitis* are ingested but not killed. Nonphagocytic cells are also involved in the immune response mechanism, for instance natural killer cells which bind to the fungus and kill through the production of toxic substances (Murphy, 1991).

Acquired immunity may arise when the fungal antigen stimulates the production of antibodies in the bloodstream. The presence of fungus-specific antibodies in the bloodstream can be used to determine exposure to a mycopathogen and the possibility of disease. Whether antibody production is necessarily protective, however, is questionable as, for example, antibody titres are often higher in those with candidiasis than in controls, and increase in patients with leukaemia dying of candidiasis. *Candida albicans* and *Cryptococcus neoformans* can, in any case, secrete proteases which may digest immunoglobulins. Nevertheless, some antibodies to *C. neoformans* may be protective and prolong survival of the patients. Suggestions are that antibodies may protect by improving phagocytosis, neutralizing the effect of enzymes responsible for the virulence of infective agents, and reducing the adhesive ability of fungal elements (Cassadevall, 1995). At the present time there is no agreed position on the function of antibody production in mycotic infections of humans.

5.3   The range of mycoses

From a practical point of view, and for convenience, mycoses are often considered in the categories cutaneous, subcutaneous, systemic and opportunistic irrespective of the mycopathogen. No attention is paid to the taxonomic group to which the mycopathogen belongs. Cutaneous, subcutaneous and systemic refer to positions in the body, whereas the opportunistic mycoses relate to fungi which are not normally expected to infect, but do so as the opportunity presents itself. Opportunistic is a teleological term and adventitious may be more appropriate, but the former is retained here as it is in almost universal usage. Although a mycopathogen may be recorded predominantly in one of the above categories, it may not necessarily be restricted to a single category. *Trichosporon beigelii*, for example, the causal agent of white piedra of the skin seen in patients in tropical and subtropical areas is, together with other species of *Trichosporon*, increasingly implicated in systemic infections in immunocompromised individuals as trichosporonosis (Table 5.2). Symptoms of aspergillosis and candidiasis can be cutaneous, subcutaneous and systemic and the organisms involved can also act as opportunists. A range of mycoses is outlined in Table 5.2.

5.3.1   *Cutaneous mycoses*

Mycoses may be superficial as in black piedra of the scalp (*Piedraia hortae*) characterized by hard black nodules on the hair shaft, and white piedra of facial hair shafts (*Trichosporon beigelii, T. ovoides*) and genital hair (*T. inkin*) characterized by soft white nodules along the hair. Pityriasis versicolour (*Malassezia furfur*) grows on superficial keratin of the skin and causes yellow to brown scaly patches on the body. *Malassezia furfur* may be implicated in the production of dandruff (seborrhoeic dermatitis), the fungus apparently

Table 5.3 Cutaneous mycoses

Syndrome	Mycopathogen
Tinea barbae (beard ringworm)	*T. mentagrophytes, T. verrucosum*
Tinea capitis (scalp ringworm)	*M. canis, T. tonsurans, T. schoenleinii*
Tinea corporis (body ringworm)	*E. floccosum, Microsporon, Trichophyton*
Tinea cruris (groin ringworm)	*E. floccosum, T. rubrum*
Tinea manuum (hand ringworm)	*E. floccosum, T. rubrum, T. mentagrophytes*
Tinea pedis (athlete's foot)	*E. floccosum, T. mentagrophytes, T. rubrum*
Tinea unguium (nail ringworm)	*T. mentagrophytes, T. rubrum*
Tinea versicolour (pityriasis)	*Malassezia furfur*

requiring sebum for growth and being unaffected by any fungicidal element in the secretion. A severe cutaneous mycosis is lobomycosis (*Loboa loboi*) which affects exposed parts of the body of people living in the Amazon area of Brazil and other Latin Amercian countries. The nodular lesions developed are very disfiguring and may require excision as drugs appear to be ineffective. Onychomycosis may be due to a range of mycopathogens including species of *Aspergillus, Candida, Onychocola,* and dermatophytes, such as *Trichophyton.* Toe and finger nails become discoloured and misshapen and the nail bed thickens, accumulates debris below, and may become difficult to cut with scissors. The main genera involved in ringworm infections of the skin are *Epidermophyton, Microsporum* and *Trichophyton* and examples are provided in Table 5.3.

Ringworm

Dermatophytes which cause mycotic infections of skin, hair and nails are confined to the keratinous (dead) layer of the skin. Dermatophytoses are worldwide, and probably account for the majority of fungal infections, occurring in people of all ages. Infection occurs when infective propagules enter minute abrasions in the keratinous layer and germinate there. Mycelium grows radially from the point of infection. An inflammatory reaction develops at the margin of the expanding, itchy lesion whilst the central zone heals. Ringworm refers to the ring-like appearance of the lesion, supposedly due to parasitic worms before it was realized that fungi were involved. Ringworm infections may spread through direct contact with an infected person (anthropophilic) or animal (zoophilic) or from spore-infested fomites. In farming communities infection may be by direct contact with infected animals, especially cattle, for instance tinea barbae, or from material infested with fungal spores. Cats, dogs, rabbits and other animals, wild, stray or domestic, can also provide a reservoir of infection although they are difficult to screen because they may not show symptoms of the disease. Parents of young children should be aware of this as the zoophilic *Microsporum canis* responsible for tinea capitis often affects children, occurring less frequently after puberty. Reasons advanced for the reduced incidence of tinea capitis in adults are improved hygiene, endocrine changes and less frequent association with the infective propagules (Bergus and Johnson, 1993). Further, sebaceous glands become active at puberty and *M. canis* is known to be sensitive to sebum (Marchisio *et al.*, 1996).

Scalp infection by *Trichophyton schoenleinii, T. violaceum* and *Microsporum gypseum* results in a chronic disease, tinea favosa, with characteristic lesions. Initial lesions comprise small red scaly patches which soon become covered by yellow crusts or scutula. The crusts are pierced by dry, lustreless hair. Crusts then coalesce to form ugly patches, hair follicles are destroyed and alopecia may result. Tinea cruris may prevail where people live in overcrowded conditions where spread appears to be associated with sharing infested fomites such as towels, bedclothes and footwear, usually in conjunction with poor hygiene. Tinea pedis, the commonest form of ringworm infection, is virtually unknown in communities where people walk barefoot. Footwear prevents feet from drying and cooling and an implication is that the warm, moist, macerating keratinous environment that fungus-infested footwear can provide may predispose towards athlete's foot. Evidence indicates that people with closed interdigital spaces where the toes are in contact suffer a significantly higher incidence of tinea pedis than those with spaces between the toes (Noguchi *et al.*, 1995). Tinea pedis infection is often accompanied by tinea manuum, perhaps due to handling fungus-infested dirty socks and shoes or using contaminated communal washing facilities. Usually, only one hand is infected (Bergus and Johnson, 1993). Although *Trichophyton rubrum* is usually regarded as responsible for ringworm infections, in the immunocompromised host the fungus may become invasive and be responsible for subcutaneous abscesses (Novick *et al.*, 1987).

5.3.2 *Subcutaneous mycoses*

Subcutaneous mycoses are caused by soil, coprophilous and entomogenous fungi and their pathogenicity is usually, although not always, limited to the cutaneous and subcutaneous tissues. Infection generally occurs through implantation of the infectious agent through the skin or mucocutaneous surface via scratches or wounds or some traumatic injury, or through inhalation of infective conidia.

Entomophthoromycosis

Entomophthoromycosis is a chronic, granulomatous inflammatory illness with two clinically distinct forms according to the causal agent, mostly occurring in the tropical areas of Africa, Asia, India, Indonesia and Latin America, although cases are known from the USA and Australia. Rhinofacial entomophthoromycosis is caused by the entomogenous *Conidiobolus coronatus* (Figure 5.1) and subcutaneous phycomycosis by *Basidiobolus* species, such as *B. haptosporus*, *B. meristosporus* and *B. ranarum* (Figure 5.1). The pathogens produce conidiospores (ballistospores) which are forcibly discharged into turbulent air. Although the precise infection mechanism is not known, it seems likely that inhaled conidiospores of *Conidiobolus* germinate on the nasal mucosa, the rapidly growing mycelium effecting entrance to the tissues through minute abrasions in the mucosal lining. With *Basidiobolus* species, the granulomas develop mainly on the trunk and limbs suggesting that they are more likely to be wound-infecting mycopathogens.

Rhinofacial entomophthoromycosis is a chronic illness in which nasal polyps develop, the paranasal sinuses are invaded and massive subcutaneous involvement of the nose and facial tissues and upper lip may occur. This mycosis is painful and disfiguring, but not usually life-threatening, although it may take years to resolve, sometimes spontaneously. The pathogen causes nasal congestion, tissue necrosis and erodes the cheekbones and orbit.

In subcutaneous phycomycosis firm, flat, moveable, indolent, slowly developing granulomas usually form in the shoulders, trunk, legs and buttocks and do not involve the underlying musculature. The maxillary sinus and hard palate may also be involved intially. The pathogen may disseminate through the lymphatic system to other parts of the body, such as the lungs, liver, muscles, pericardium, stomach and colon, and be life-threatening. Microabscesses are scattered throughout the infected tissues.

Sporotrichosis

The causal agent *Sporothrix schenckii*, basically a wound pathogen, causes chronic subcutaneous lymphomycosis resulting from accidental implantation of the fungus into subcutaneous tissue when the skin of the limbs and face is punctured by mycelium/spore-infested splinters of wood, thorns or other plant debris. Sporotrichosis occurs most frequently amongst plant nursery employees, home gardeners, florists and agricultural workers, especially when previously exposed to *Sphagnum* (moss), and miners exposed to splinters from pit props. Infection in humans has also been associated with bites, pecks and stings inflicted by various animals including rodents, cats, dogs, horses, chickens and a boa constrictor, and those handling contaminated plant materials such as timber and mosses or tropical fish (Frean *et al.*, 1991). Inhalation of dust from *Sphagnum* can result in acute respiratory infection (Agger *et al.*, 1985). Zoonotic transmission from a badly infected cat to a veterinary surgeon appears to have involved exposure to a massive inoculum without associated wounding (Reed *et al.*, 1992). Sporotrichosis is mainly tropical although cases have also been reported in America, Japan and France.

Sporothrix schenckii is dimorphic (Figure 5.2), the saprobic conidial M-phase growing in association with plant materials in soil, the budding Y-phase in the tissues where over 80 per cent of the yeast cells may be associated with characteristic asteroidal bodies. About 3 weeks after infection, either a small painless ulcer which fails to heal develops at the inoculation site, or a pink subcutaneous nodule arises which eventually adheres to the overlying skin and then ulcerates. The infection then enters the dermal lymphatic system and produces chronic nodular lymphomycosis. The nodules slowly enlarge, eventually undergo necrosis and discharge pus into the lymph. Related lymph nodes may also enlarge. The lesions may persist for years if untreated and sometimes the infection disseminates producing lesions in the skin, lungs, kidneys, testes, limb joints, bones, eyes and meninges. Treatment of the subcutaneous infection with an oral saturated solution of potassium iodide is usually successful although the patient may not be able to tolerate the side effects. The application of liquid nitrogen, however, dries lesions and can result in complete healing (Bargman, 1995). Heat treatment, and itraconazole taken orally, are also effective (Kaufman, 1992).

Maduramycosis

Maduramycosis (mycetoma or Madura foot) is a chronic infection of the cutaneous and subcutaneous tissues, usually of the hands and feet, caused by various actinomycetes and fungi in the tropics. Some of the mycopathogens involved are *Madurella grisea*, *M. mycetomatis*, *Pseudallescheria boydii*, *Leptosphaeria senegalensis*, *Aspergillus* and *Phialophora* species and *Fusarium solani*. Infection occurs when the hand or foot is penetrated by a fungus-contaminated thorn or splinter. The mycopathogens, which grow slowly in the tissues, cause localized enlargement of the infection site from which pus containing characteristically coloured granules, according to the type of pathogen, is exuded. *Madurella* species and *F. solani* are responsible for black-dot mycetoma and in aspergillotic mycetoma the mycotic grains are usually white to yellow. With *F. solani* numerous papules develop around the infection site, which enlarge and form draining sinuses (Thianprasit and Sivayathorn, 1983). Response to antifungal antibiotics is usually poor and lesions may have to be excised. The disease progresses slowly, is disfiguring through deformation of the affected area, and eventually involves bones of the limb which may require amputation.

5.3.3 *Systemic mycoses*

Infective propagules of systemic mycopathogens are often inhaled and the disease which may begin as a secondary lung infection disseminates to other parts of the body via the bloodstream, lymphatic system and cerebrospinal fluid. In dimorphic systemic pathogens it is usually the Y-phase which is pathogenic, although the M-phase predominates in systemic *Candida* infections of the tissues.

Aspergillosis

Aspergillus species grow rapidly and sporulate profusely in decaying fermenting compost heaps, hay stored in damp decaying vegetation and on cereal grains and other foods stored under warm damp conditions, all of which provide a reservoir of allergenic and infective spores. Several species of *Aspergillus* (Figure 5.1) are involved in the various manifestations of aspergillosis although *A. fumigatus*, *A. flavus* and *A. niger* appear to predominate. Inhaled conidiospores grow in the abscess cavities of lungs already weakened through a primary infection such as pneumonia or tuberculosis. Mycelium may fill the cavities producing aspergillomas or fungus balls which provide continuous exposure to the allergens and potentially invasive hyphae and infective spores. *Aspergillus* pneumonia may develop in patients receiving cytotoxic or immunosuppressive therapy and the organism may disseminate to the skin, brain, eyes, heart, gastrointestinal tract, kidneys, cartilage, bone and elsewhere.

Disseminated aspergillosis is invariably coupled with underlying illness in the immunocompromised and is often fatal. Invasion of blood vessels with necrotic areas (infarctions) characterizes pneumonic and disseminated infection.

Blastomycosis

Blastomyces dermatidis (Figure 5.2), the causal agent of North American blastomycosis, is dimorphic with a conidial M-phase, probably surviving saprobically in soil, and a budding intracellular Y-phase in the tissues. Blastomycosis is endemic in the Great Lakes region of the USA and Canada. Infection appears to occur either through inhalation of airborne conidiospores resulting in an initial lung infection or by penetration of the infective agent through wounds in the skin. The chronic granulomatous, suppurative disease which can be fatal, disseminates haematogenously, especially in immunocompromised patients, mainly to the skin but can also involve the bones, joints, larynx, prostate gland, central nervous and urinogenital systems.

Candidiasis (moniliasis, candidosis)

Candidiasis, due to the dimorphic yeast *Candida albicans* (Figure 5.2) and other pathogenic species, usually develops on mucous membranes forming cream-white lesions in mucocutaneous oral thrush and vulvovaginitis. *Candida* species are usually constituents of the normal body microflora and may be isolated from the mucous membranes, hand and elsewhere on the skin, sputum, bronchial washings, faeces and urine. The yeast is transmitted between individuals by contact with mouth and vaginal fluids, skin excretions, and faeces, especially from patients or carriers, and can also be passed from mother to baby during childbirth. Systemic candidiasis develops from mucosal lesions, use of unsterile hypodermic syringes in drug addicts, intravenous catheters and catheters in the bladder of patients with urinary disorders and serious burns. In AIDS, cancer and other immunocompromised patients, ulcers form in the oesophagus, gastrointestinal tract and bladder; haematogenous dissemination may result in lesions in kidneys, lungs, liver, heart, eye, meninges and brain and on the skin. Pulmonary mycetoma due to *C. albicans* has also been recognized (Shelley *et al.*, 1996). The M-phase, comprising hyphae and pseudomycelial elements, tends to predominate in infected tissues and the budding Y-phase cells in body fluids, although both phases are usually present.

Cryptococcosis (torulosis)

Cryptococcus neoformans is an encapsulated budding yeast (Figure 5.1) associated with vegetable matter in soil and the faeces of pigeons and other birds which are not themselves infected but may also carry the pathogen on their feet and beaks. The fungus assimilates creatinine found in bird droppings. If dried droppings are disturbed mechanically, for example by people walking over them or in cleaning bird cages, yeast cells and particulate matter carrying the infective agent, which may also include dried basidiospores of the teleomorph *Filobasidiella neoformans*, enter the atmosphere and may be inhaled. Primary nodular lesions develop in the lungs and in severely immunocompromised people the disease spreads via the bloodstream primarily to the central nervous system. Dissemination to the skin, prostate glands, eyes and bones can also occur. Cryptococcosis is a major cause of meningitis in patients with AIDS and the yeast may be isolated from the cerebrospinal fluid.

Coccidiomycosis

Coccidiomycosis, caused by the dimorphic mycopathogen *Coccidiodes immitis* (Figure 5.2), appears limited to the western hemisphere, being endemic in the southern USA and South America. In the saprobic phase in the soil the mycelium produces chains of thick-walled arthrospores which are inhaled and may initiate lung infection. Arthrospores within the lung swell and transform into characteristic thick-walled spherules containing masses of units referred to as endospores. Breakdown of spherules releases endospores which enlarge to form further spherules, so continuing the infection. Although arthrospores are highly infectious, rapid spontaneous recovery from the pulmonary infection with influenza-like symptoms is said to occur in over 99 per cent of cases and such patients appear immune to further infection from *C. immitis*. Serious systemic illness which can be fatal, however, occurs in the minority of cases where abscesses containing spherules develop in the meninges, thyroid gland, joints, bones and subcutaneous tissues.

Histoplasmosis

North American histoplasmosis, caused by the dimorphic *Histoplasma capsulatum* (Figure 5.2), occurs mainly in the Ohio and Mississippi regions of the USA. African histoplamosis is caused by *H. duboisii*. The M-phase of

H. capsulatum which produces microconidia and macro-conidia lives saprobically in soil, and in association with faeces of chickens, and bird and bat roosting sites. Inhalation of the conidiospores results in an initial lung infection. The intracellular budding yeast phase of the disease, initially respiratory and then systemic, may progress rapidly throughout the lymph system to form granulomatous ulcerating lesions of the lips, gums, tongue, larynx and throat. The progressive disseminated disease can be fatal.

5.3.4　*Opportunistic mycopathogens*

Any fungus capable of growing at 37°C should be regarded as a potential opportunistic pathogen, thus this category includes cutaneous, subcutaneous and systemic mycopathogens. Many opportunistic mycoses, however, are those reported for the first time, such as *Rhizopus azygosporus* in premature babies (Schipper *et al.*, 1996). Opportunistic mycopathogens causing fungaemia or affecting particular parts of the body are increasingly responsible for disease. The same predisposing factors apply to opportunistic mycopathogens as to other categories of mycoses. Opportunistic mycoses present a risk especially for the immunocompromised with underlying debilitating illness requiring chemotherapy and the extensive use of antibiotics, particularly multiple antibacterial antibiotics. Many fungi not previously thought of as human pathogens have recently joined the increasing list of mycotic agents and these have been referred to as emerging pathogens (Perfect and Schell, 1996; Rossman *et al.*, 1996). The most frequent nosocomial (hospital-acquired) mycosis in patients with AIDS is candidiasis, and about 7 per cent of patients develop cryptococcosis. Approximately 8–10 per cent of nosocomial infections are mycoses and of those about 80 per cent are due to *Candida* species (Bullock *et al.*, 1993), often causing fungaemia. Nosocomial *Candida* infections may spread from patient to patient through personal contact or contact with contaminated fomites. Hospital personnel may carry the yeast on their hands and provide a potential source of infection. The frequency of nosocomial candidiasis has increased markedly during the 1980s and 1990s (Pfaller, 1995, 1996) and many species of *Candida* in addition to *C. albicans* appear to be increasingly involved. Several other opportunistic mycopathogens cause nosocomial fungaemia, for example *Fusarium oxysporum*, and the yeasts *Kluyveromyces marxianus*, *Lodderomyces elongisporus*, *Rhodotorula glutinis*, *R. minuta*, *R. rubra*, *Saccharomyces cerevisiae* and *Pichia anomala*, usually associated with the removal of intravascular catheters.

Accidental inoculation of the body in the laboratory has resulted in opportunistic infections of blastomycosis, coccidiomycosis, cryptococcosis, histoplasmosis and sporotrichosis (Sewell, 1995), and the intentional intravenous injection by drug abusers of lemon or orange juice, excellent growth media for *Candida* species, in candidiasis. Nosocomial aspergillosis mostly due to *A. fumigatus*, correlated apparently with ventilation systems where conidiospores may accumulate, or dust associated with building work, sometimes occurs (Bodey and Vartivarian, 1989).

Zygomycosis (mucormycosis, phycomycosis)

Several members of the Mucorales (Figure 5.3) are opportunistic pathogens and the disease syndrome is broadly referred to as zygomycosis (Table 5.2). Over 95 per cent of reported cases of zygomycoses involve people with diabetes, immunosuppression, debilitating disease such as tuberculosis or severe burns; rarely is it associated with AIDS. Opportunism is exemplified by various forms of trauma associated with zygomycosis, for example vehicle accidents; tattoos (e.g. *Saksenaea vasiformis*); arterial, venous, bladder and peritoneal cathetization (e.g. *Rhizopus* sp.); skin injury (e.g. *Apophysomyces elegans*); spider bite (*Rhizopus* spp.); abdominal surgery, bone marrow transplantation; and in association with the use of desferrioxamine in renal dialysis patients. Primary zygomycosis although infrequent is, nevertheless, serious causing for example osteomyelitis necessitating limb amputation (*A. elegans, S. vasiformis*), invasive cutaneous zygomycosis (*S. vasiformis, Syncephalastrum racemosum*) and rhinocerebral zygomycosis (*S. vasiformis*). Rhinocerebral, central nervous system and osteomyelytic zygomycoses (e.g. *Absidia corymbifera, Rhizopus arrhizus, R. oryzae*) are usually associated with diabetes mellitus, lymphomas and cirrhosis of the liver. Gastrointestinal zygomycosis may be associated with malnutrition, uraemia (blood in the urine), kwashiorkor (illness due to lack of protein in the diet) and liver transplantation. Pulmonary and disseminated zygomycosis may accompany haematological malignancies and diabetes mellitus (e.g. *Absidia corymbifera, Cunninghamella bertholletiae, Mucor circinelloides*). Postoperative cutaneous zygomycosis (*Rhizopus* spp.), which may strike after the application of contaminated adhesive plaster dressings, causes ulceration which can extend to the subcutaneous tissues. Endocarditis and vascular zygomycosis may follow surgery involving coronary artery bypass, heart valve replacement and organ transplantation (e.g. *C. bertholletiae*).

Inhalation and entry of the sporangiospores through the nasal mucosa is the usual means of ingress, although any break in the skin or mucocutaneous lining is sufficient for entry of the pathogen. In rhinocerebral zygomycosis, hyphae grow through the paranasal sinuses and orbit to the brain. Invasion of blood vessels with necrosis of surrounding tissues occurs. The disease is normally rapidly progressive and destructive, fulminant (exploding) and usually fatal unless early identification is made and treatment undertaken. Hyphae which initially invade and occlude the lumina of the arteries induce thrombosis, and are responsible for necrosis of the surrounding tissues. Lymphatic and venous invasion occurs after initial arterial colonization. A nutritional requirement for iron may explain the predilection for growth in blood vessels. The fungus grows in the necrotic tissue and extends rapidly along the injured blood vessels (Brown and Finn, 1986). Haematogenous spread results in systemic zygomycosis which affects many parts of the body, such as the brain, lungs, kidneys and liver. Characteristically the hyphae, frequently observed at autopsy, are broad, non-septate and readily recognizable although growth in culture is necessary for generic and specific identification of the pathogen to be made.

Zygomycosis may be treated with the antifungal antibiotic liposomal amphotericin B and surgical debridement of necrotic areas coupled with treatment of underlying medical problems. Amphotericin resistance is known, however, and various chemotherapeutic drugs, such as azoles, are also used to combat this and many other forms of mycotic illness. Vascular thrombosis prevents amphotericin B from reaching the fungus in the necrotic tissues, thus surgical debridement removes a region of infection that cannot be adequately treated with systemic medication alone. In diabetes mellitus, ketotic acidosis increases susceptibility to infection by reducing the phagocytic ability of granulocytes and the serum also has a reduced immunological ability to combat the fungus.

5.3.5 *Other opportunistic mycotic fungi*

In patients with AIDS some cutaneous infections (e.g. *Alternaria* spp., *Paracoccidioides brasiliensis*), brain abscesses (*Aureobasidium pullulans*), pneumonia (*Fusarium* spp., *Pneumocystis carinii*), meningitis (*Cryptococcus neoformans*) and disseminated infections (*P. brasiliensis*, *Penicillium decumbens*, *Scedosporium inflatum*) are opportunistic mycoses (Kaplan *et al.*, 1995). Blastomycosis, histoplasmosis and coccidiomycosis also occur in patients with AIDS in areas where these mycoses are endemic (Wheat, 1995). Several opportunistic mycopathogens invade the central nervous system including species of *Alternaria*, *Cephalosporium*, *Curvularia*, *Geotrichum*, *Paecilomyces* and *Schizophyllum*. *Phialophora repens*, a lignicolous saprobe, is now known also to cause subcutaneous phaeohyphomycosis (Hironaga *et al.*, 1989), and *Exserohilum longirostratum* sight-threatening corneal ulcers (Bouchon *et al.*, 1994). Although fungi are not normally components of the microflora of the eye, the spectrum of opportunistic mycopathogens responsible for fungal keratitis in contact lens wearers is wide, including both yeasts and filamentous moulds. The literature now abounds with examples of emerging opportunistic mycoses, which also serves to emphasize the caution required when coming into close contact with fungi.

Summary

- Mycopathogens of humans occur worldwide and are known from all of the main groups of fungi. The infectious agents may be acquired through direct contact with the skin and mucocutaneous surfaces, inhaled, ingested, enter the body when damaged accidentally or through some surgical procedures. Any tissue or organ in the body may become infected, especially in the severely immunocompromised.

- Components of walls of the M-phase and Y-phase of mycopathogens may be antigenic. Virulence factors expressed during the pathogenic phase of growth include a range of extracellular digestive enzymes which facilitate growth in tissue, and adhesive properties enabling cells to stick fast to mucocutaneous surfaces. The production of antibiotics, secondary metabolites and capsular material may augment the process of infection by certain mycopathogens.

- Mycoses tend to be either cutaneous, subcutaneous or systemic, although in immunocompromised hosts, particularly those suffering from AIDS and underlying malignant illnesses, the effects of a single mycosis such as candidiasis may present in more than one of those categories. A range of factors believed to predispose the host to infection is considered.

- Any fungus capable of growing at body temperature should be regarded as a potential opportunistic pathogen. Many opportunistic mycopathogens, the emerging pathogens, causing fungaemia or affecting particular parts of the body are increasingly responsible for infections in immunocompromised patients requiring chemotherapy and the extensive use of antibiotics.

Study problems

1. With reference to named examples distinguish between:
   (i)   the saprobic and parasitic modes of life,
   (ii)   the Y-phase and M-phase of growth,
   (iii) Basidiomycota and Zygomycota,
   (iv)   primary and secondary mycoses.
2. Explain how hyphae and sporulation structures may assist the physician in the identification of mycopathogens.
3. Outline the factors which may predispose individuals to fungal infections.
4. Using named examples of mycotic agents define the following terms:
   (i)   nosocomial mycosis,
   (ii)   subcutaneous mycosis,
   (iii) candidiasis,
   (iv)   aspergillosis.
5. Summarize possible mechanisms of immunity to mycoses.

Selected reading

Agger, W.A., La Crosse, W.I. and Seager, G.M., 1985, Granulomas of the vocal cords caused by *Sporothrix schenckii*, *Laryngoscope*, **95**, 595–596

Ahearn, D.G. and Price, D.L., 1995, Fungi in hospital environments, *Clin. Microbiol. Updates*, **7**, 1–6

Ahmad, M., Dar, M.A., Weinstein, A.J., Mehta, A.C. and Golish, J.A., 1984, Thoracic aspergillosis (Part II), *Cleveland Clinic Quarterly*, **51**, 631–653

Ajello, L., 1956, Soil as natural reservoir for human pathogenic fungi, *Science*, **123**, 876–879

Andersen, P., Schonheyder, H. and Oster, S., 1985, Primary pulmonary aspergillosis. A case study, *Mykosen*, **28**, 595–598

Arruda, L.K., Muir, A., Vailes, L.D., Selden, R.F., Platts-Mills, T.A.E. and Chapman, M.D., 1995, Antibody responses to *Aspergillus fumigatus* allergens in patients with cystic fibrosis, *Int. Arch. Allergy Immunol.*, **107**, 410–411

Bargman, H., 1995, Successful treatment of cutaneous sporotrichosis with liquid nitrogen: report of three cases, *Mycoses*, **38**, 285–287

Bergus, G.R. and Johnson, J.S., 1993, Superficial tinea infections, *Am. Fam. Physician*, **48**, 259–268

Binazzi, M., Papini, M. and Simonetti, S., 1983, Skin mycoses – geographic distribution and present-day pathomorphosis, *Int. J. Dermatol.*, **22**, 92–97

Bodey, G.P. and Vartivarian, S., 1989, Aspergillosis, *Eur. J. Clin. Microbiol. Infect. Dis.*, **8**, 413–437

Bouchon, C.L., Greer, D.L. and Genre, C.F., 1994, Corneal ulcer due to *Exserohilum longirostratum*, *Clin. Microbiol. Infect. Dis.*, **101**, 452–455

Brown, O.E. and Finn, R., 1986, Mucormycosis of the mandible, *J. Oral Maxillofac. Surg.*, **44**, 132–136

Bullock, W., Kozel, T., Scherer, S. and Dixon, D.M., 1993, Medical mycology in the 1990s: involvement of NIH and the wider community, *ASM News*, **59**, 182–185

Cailliez, J.C., Seguy, N., Denis, C.M., Aliouat, E.M., Mazars, E., Polonelli, L., Camus, D. and Dei-Cas, E., 1996, *Pneumocystis carinii*: an atypical fungal micro-organism, *J. Med. Vet. Mycol.*, **34**, 227–239

Cassadevall, A., 1995, Antibody immunity and invasive fungal infections, *Infect. Immun.*, **63**, 4211–4218

Chandler, F.W., Watts, J.C., Kaplan, W., Hendry, A.T., McGinnis, M.R. and Ajello, L., 1985, Zygomycosis. Report of four cases with formation of chlamydoconidia in tissue, *Am. J. Clin. Pathol.*, **84**, 99–103

English, M.P., 1980, *Medical Mycology*, The Institute of Biology's Studies in Biology No. 119: Edward Arnold, 57 pp

Fenelon, L., 1997, Unusual infections and new diagnostic methods in the immunocompromised host, *Curr. Opin. Infect. Dis.*, **10**, 285–288

Ferrinho, P.del G.M., 1985, Pulmonary phycomycosis without obvious predisposing factors, *S. African Med. J.*, **68**, 893

Frank, K.A., Merz, W.G. and Hutchins, G.M., 1988, Sclerotium formation in an *Aspergillus flavus* wound infection, *Mycopathologia*, **102**, 185–188

Frean, J.A., Isaacson, M., Miller, G.B., Mistry, B.D. and Heney, C., 1991, Sporotrichosis following a rodent bite, *Mycopathologia*, **116**, 5–8

Goldani, L.Z., Craven, D.E. and Sugar, A.M., 1995, Central venous catheter infection with *Rhodotorula minuta* in a patient with AIDS taking suppressive doses of fluconazole, *J. Med. Vet. Mycol.*, **33**, 267–270

Harrell, E. and Curtis, A.C., 1959, North American blastomycosis, *Am. J. Med.*, **21**, 750–766

Hawksworth, D.L., Kirk, P.M., Sutton, B.C. and Pegler, D.N., 1995, *Ainsworth & Bisby's Dictionary of the Fungi*, Wallingford: CAB International, 616 pp

Hironaga, M., Nakano, K., Yokoyama, I. and Kitajina, J., 1989, *Phialophora repens*, an emerging agent of subcutaneous phaeohyphomycosis in humans, *J. Clin. Microbiol.*, **27**, 394–399

Horner, W.E., Helbling, J.E., Salvaggio, J.E. and Lehrer, S.B., 1995, Fungal allergens, *Clin. Microbiol. Rev.*, **8**, 161–179

Howard, D.H., 1984, The epidemiology and ecology of blastomycosis, coccidiomycosis and histoplasmosis, *Zentralblatt fuer Bakteriologie, Parasitenkunde, Infektionshrankheiten und Hygiene, Series A*, **257**, 219–227

Jeffries, P. and Young, T.W.K., 1983, Light and electron microscopy of vegetative hyphae, septum formation, and yeast-mould dimorphism in *Cokeromyces recurvatus*, *Protoplasma*, **117**, 206–213

Jeffries, P. and Young, T.W.K., 1994, *Interfungal Parasitic Relationships*, Wallingford: CAB International, 296 pp

Kaplan, J.E., Masur, H., Holmes, K.J., McNeil, M.M., Schonberger, L.B., Navin, T.R., Hanson, D.L., Gross, P.A., Jaffe, H.W. and the USPHS/IDSA Prevention of Opportunistic Infections Working Group, 1995, *Clin. Infect. Dis.*, **21**, S1–S11

Kaufman, L., 1992, Laboratory methods for the diagnosis and confirmation of systemic mycoses, *Clin. Infect. Dis.*, **14**, S23–S29

Kemna, M.E., Neri, R.C., Ali, R. and Salkin, I.F., 1994, *Cokeromyces recurvatus*, a mucoraceous zygomycete rarely isolated in clinical laboratories, *J. Clin. Microbiol.*, **32**, 843–845

Kennedy, M.J., Rogers, A.L., Laurey, R., Hanselmen, D.R., Soll, D.R. and Yancey, R.J., 1988, Variation in adhesion and cell surface hydrophobicity in *Candida albicans* white and opaque phenotypes, *Mycopathologia*, **102**, 149–156

Kheir, S.M., Flint, A. and Moss, J., 1983, Primary aspergillosis of the larynx simulating carcinoma, *Hum. Pathol.*, **14**, 184–186

Kiehn, T.E., Gorey, E., Brown, A.E., Edwards, F.F. and Armstrong, D., 1992, Sepsis due to *Rhodotorula* related to use of indwelling central venous catheters, *Clin. Infect. Dis.*, **14**, 841–846

Kwon-Chung, K.J., 1994, Phylogenetic spectrum of fungi that are pathogenic to humans, *Clin. Infect. Dis.*, **19**, S1–S7

Lacey, J., 1991, Aerobiology and health: the role of airborne fungal spores in respiratory disease, in Hawksworth, D.L. (ed.) *Frontiers in Mycology*, Wallingford: CAB International, pp. 157–185

Leu, H.-S., Lee, A.Y.-S. and Kuo, T.-T., 1995, Recurrence of *Fusarium solani* abscess formation in an otherwise healthy patient, *Infection*, **23**, 303/53–305/55

Mahe, A., Develoux, M., Lienhardt, C., Keita, S. and Bobin, P., 1996, Mycetomas in Mali: causative agents and geographic distribution, *Am. J. Trop. Med.*, **54**, 77–79

Male, O., 1991, The significance of mycology in medicine, in Hawksworth, D.L. (ed.) *Frontiers in Mycology*, Wallingford: CAB International, pp. 131–156

Manfredi, R., Mazzoni, A., Nanetti, A. and Chiodo, F., 1994, Histoplasmosis capsulati and duboissi in Europe, *Eur. J. Epidemiol.*, **10**, 1–7

Marchisio, V.F., Preve, L. and Tullio, V., 1996, Fungi responsible for skin mycoses in Turin (Italy), *Mycoses*, **39**, 141–150

Murphy, J.W., 1986, Host defenses against pathogenic fungi, *Clin. Immunol. Newslett.*, **7**, 17–22

Murphy, J.W., 1991, Mechanisms of natural resistance to human pathogenic fungi, *Annu. Rev. Microbiol.*, **45**, 509–538

Musial, C.E., Cockerill III, F.R. and Roberts, G.D., 1988, Fungal infections of the immunocompromised host: clinical and laboratory aspects, *Clin. Microbiol. Rev.*, **1**, 349–364

Noguchi, H., Hiruma, M., Kawada, A., Ishibashi, A. and Kono, S., 1995, Tinea pedis in members of the Japanese self-defence forces: relationships of its prevalence and its severity with length of military service and width of interdigital spaces, *Mycoses*, **38**, 495–499

Novick, N.L., Tapia, L. and Bottone, E.J., 1987, Invasive *Trichophyton rubrum* infection in an immunocompromised host, *Am. J. Med.*, **82**, 321–325

Pegler, D.N. and Young, T.W.K., 1971, *Basidiospore morphology in the Agaricales*, Lehre, Germany: J. Cramer, 210 pp

Perfect, J.R. and Schell, W.A., 1996, The new fungal opportunists are coming, *Clin. Infect. Dis.*, **22**, S112–S118

Pfaller, M.A., 1995, Epidemiology of candidiasis, *J. Hosp. Infect.*, **30**, 329–338

Pfaller, M.A., 1996, Nosocomial candidiasis: emerging species, reservoirs, and modes of transmission, *Clin. Infect. Dis.*, **22**, S89–S94

Raad, I. and Hachem, R., 1995, Treatment of central venous catheter-related fungemia due to *Fusarium oxysporum*, *Clin. Infect. Dis.*, **20**, 709–711

Reed, K.D., Moore, F.M., Geiger, G.E. and Stemper, M.E., 1992, Zoonotic transmission of sporotrichosis: case report and review, *Clin. Infect. Dis.*, **16**, 384–387

Restrepo, A., Salazar, M.E., Cano, L.E., Stover, E.P., Feldman, D. and Stevens, D.A., 1984, Estrogens inhibit mycelium-to-yeast transformation in the fungus *Paracoccidioides brasiliensis*: implications for resistance of females to paracoccidiomycosis, *Infect. Immun.*, **46**, 346–353

Rihs, J.D., Padhye, A.A. and Good, C.B., 1996, Brain abscess caused by *Schizophyllum commune*: an emerging basidiomycete pathogen, *J. Clin. Microbiol.*, **34**, 1628–1632

Rossman, S.N., Cernoch, P.L. and Davis, J.R., 1996, Dematiaceous fungi are an increasing cause of human disease, *Clin. Infect. Dis.*, **22**, 73–80

San-Blas, G., 1982, The cell wall of fungal human pathogens: its possible role in host-parasite relationships, *Mycopathologia*, **79**, 159–184

Schipper, M.A.A., Maslen, M.M., Hogg, G.G., Chow, C.W. and Samson, R.A., 1996, Human infection by *Rhizopus azygosporus* and the occurrence of azygospores in Zygomycetes, *J. Med. Vet. Mycol.*, **34**, 199–203

Seaton, A. and Robertson, M.D., 1989, *Aspergillus*, asthma and amoebae, *Lancet*, April 22, 893–894

Sewell, D.L., 1995, Laboratory-associated infections and biosafety, *Clin. Microbiol. Rev.*, **8**, 389–405

Shelley, M.A., Poe, R.H. and Kapner, L.B., 1996, Pulmonary mycetoma due to *Candida albicans*: case report and review, *Clin. Infect. Dis.*, **22**, 133–135

Stevens, D.A., 1995, Coccidiomycosis, *New Engl. J. Med.*, **332**, 1077–1082

Stringer, J.R. and Walzer, P.D., 1996, Molecular biology and epidemiology of *Pneumocystis carinii* infection in AIDS, *AIDS*, **10**, 561–571

Thianprasit, M. and Sivayathorn, A., 1983, Black dot mycetoma, *Mykosen*, **27**, 219–226

Tomee, J.F.C., Kaufman, H.F., Klimp, A.H., de Monchy, J.G.R., Koeter, G.H. and Dubois, A.E.J., 1994, Immunologic significance of a collagen-derived culture filtrate containing proteolytic activity in *Aspergillus*-related species, *J. Allergy Clin. Immunol.*, **93**, 768–778

Vainrub, B., Macareno, A., Mandel, S. and Musher, D.M., 1988, Wound zygomycosis (mucormycosis) in otherwise healthy adults, *Am. J. Med.*, **84**, 546–548

Vartivarian, S.E., 1992, Virulence properties and nonimmune pathogenic mechanisms, *Clin. Infect. Dis.*, **14**, S30–S36

Wagner, D.K. and Sohnle, P.G., 1995, Cutaneous defences against dermatophytes and yeasts, *Clin. Microbiol. Rev.*, **8**, 317–335

Wheat, J., 1995, Endemic mycoses in AIDS: a clinical review, *Clin. Microbiol. Rev.*, **8**, 146–159

Willemsen, M.J., De Coninck, A.L., Coremans-Pelseneer, J.E., Marichal-Pipeleers, M.A. and Roseeuw, D.I., 1986, Parasitic invasion of *Fusarium oxysporum* in an arterial ulcer in an otherwise healthy patient, *Mykosen*, **29**, 248–252

Young, T.W.K., 1969, Electron microscopic study of the asexual structures in Mucorales, *Proc. Linnean Soc. Lond.*, **179**, 1–9

6 Vaccines

A vaccine can be defined as an immunogenic preparation of a pathogen which engenders immunity without causing disease. A vaccine exploits the immunological phenomenon of memory (section 1.3), such that the primary exposure to the antigen in the vaccine elicits a pool of memory T and B lymphocytes that, upon subsequent exposure to the same antigen, are activated and effect clearance of the pathogen before disease occurs. In this chapter we will learn about conventional vaccine design, and how recombinant DNA technology has opened up opportunities for the production of engineered vaccines that promise to resolve several shortcomings of the conventional approaches.

6.1 Conventional vaccines

Conventional approaches to vaccine design have changed very little in the last 100 years. There are two basic approaches: **inactivation** and **attenuation** of a pathogen. Inactivation can be performed by exposure to chemical fixatives, by heat denaturation, or by exposure to irradiation. Examples are listed in Table 6.1.

As a general rule, inactivated pathogens are particularly efficient at eliciting antibodies, and are therefore useful for providing prophylactic protection, but much less effective at eliciting CD8+ cytotoxic T lymphocytes (T_C cells). Entry into the class I pathway, which is required for presentation in the context of class I HLA molecules to T_C cells, requires the antigen to be synthesized endogenously (see Figure 1.3 in Chapter 1). Nevertheless, being dead, such vaccines are relatively easy to store and refrigeration is not essential. However, non-living antigens are not particularly immunogenic and require the use of an **adjuvant** to elicit a good inflammatory reaction. Persistence of the antigen is relatively short and the immunity engendered is short term (< 10 years), so regular booster immunizations are required to maintain adequately high levels of serum antibodies. There is also the risk of under- or overinactivating the vaccine. Inadequate inactivation may leave viable pathogenic organisms or toxins in the vaccine preparation, whereas excessive denaturation may change the three-dimensional conformation of the

Table 6.1 Currently used conventional vaccines

Disease	Type[1]	Route of immunization[2]	Notes
Viruses			
Polio (Salk)	Inactivated	i.m., s.c.	Produced in monkey kidney cells, human cell lines
Influenza	Inactivated (whole or subunit)	i.m.	Antigenic variation necessitates production of new vaccine for epidemic each year; produced in hen eggs
Rabies	Inactivated	i.m.	Postexposure prophylaxis; produced originally in animal brains, now in human cell lines
Hepatitis A	Inactivated	i.m.	Produced in human cell lines
Hepatitis B	Inactivated (HBsAg subunit particle)	i.m.	Produced originally from serum of carriers, now produced in yeast; first recombinant vaccine licenced for human use
Polio (Sabin)	Attenuated	oral	The triple oral polio vaccine (OPV) comprising three main polio serotypes
Chickenpox (varicella zoster virus)	Attenuated	i.m.	
Smallpox (variola)	Attenuated (vaccinia)	scarification	Original source of vaccinia probably horse; provides protective immunity to variola virus
Measles	Attenuated	s.c., i.m.	Produced in chick embryo cells; measles vaccine often administered combined with mumps and rubella vaccines (MMR) to infants
Mumps	Attenuated	s.c., i.m.	Produced in chick embryo cells
Rubella	Attenuated	s.c., i.m.	Produced in duck or human cell lines

Bacteria		Route[2]	
		i.d., i.m., s.c.	
Cholera (*Vibrio cholerae*)	Inactivated		
Whooping cough (pertussis) (*Bordetella pertussis*)	Inactivated (whole or combined subunit)	i.m.	Subunit vaccine reportedly less toxic than whole inactivated; pertussis vaccine often administered with diphtheria and tetanus toxoids (DPT) to newborn infants
Plague (*Yersinia pestis*)	Inactivated (subunit capsular polysaccharide)	i.m.	Poor stimulator of T_H cells; therefore IgM only and no class switching to IgG; no memory
Meningococcal meningitis (*Neisseria meningitidis*)	Inactivated (subunit capsular polysaccharide)	i.m.	ditto
Pneumococcal pneumonia (*Streptococcus pneumoniae*)	Inactivated (subunit capsular polysaccharide)	i.m.	ditto
Meningitis (*Haemophilus influenzae*)	Inactivated (subunit capsular polysaccharide coupled to carrier)	i.m.	Capsular polysaccharide coupled to carrier protein (tetanus toxoid or meningococcal protein) to improve immunogenicity
Tetanus (*Clostridium tetani*)	Inactivated (subunit toxoid)	i.m.	
Diphtheria (*Corynebacterium diphtheriae*)	Inactivated (subunit toxoid)	i.m.	
Tuberculosis (*Mycobacterium tuberculosis*)	Attenuated (*M. bovis*)	i.d.	

[1] Whole organism unless otherwise stated.

[2] i.m., intramuscular; s.c., subcutaneous; i.d., intradermal.

antigen such that the antibodies elicited may fail to cross-react with the native antigen.

In contrast, attenuated vaccines are specially adapted strains of live microorganisms that retain infectivity but are non-pathogenic. Attenuation of a pathogen relies on naturally occurring variability in virulence within a given population. In practice, attenuation is a time-consuming trial and error process that is achieved by culturing pathogens in unnatural hosts or *in vitro* to select strains less adapted for growth in humans. Attenuated intracellular pathogens, such as viruses and intracellular bacteria, retain their ability to infect cells and elicit T_C-cell responses as well as antibody. Moreover, live vaccines tend to persist for longer than inactivated ones and engender longer lasting immunity without the need for repeat immunizations. An adjuvant is not normally necessary as a good live vaccine usually retains its natural inflammatory properties. The main disadvantages associated with attenuation are the ever-present risk of reversion back to virulence, and the need for cold storage which precludes their use in some countries. A few conventional vaccines are considered below.

Polio

Polio virus is acquired orally; it replicates in the mucosal epithelium of the gut and becomes released into the blood. The final target tissue is the central nervous system, leading to neural pathology and muscle paralysis. Polio virus is genetically stable (only three serotypes exist) so it is possible to confer complete protection with vaccines. The Salk polio vaccine is a formalin-inactivated preparation of all three serotypes which first underwent trials in the USA in the mid-1950s. The Salk vaccine is administered by injection and, as with all non-living vaccines, several immunizations are necessary to elicit sufficiently high titres of neutralizing antibodies. While Salk was developing the inactivated vaccine, Sabin produced attenuated strains of polio virus by repeated subculturing in monkey kidney cells *in vitro*. Variants of all three virulent serotypes were isolated that were non-virulent in monkeys but which elicited good antibody responses. The vaccine is administered orally (OPV – oral polio vaccine), usually on a sugar cube. Full immunity requires three separate doses as only one of the three strains dominates the induced response each time. These days the attenuated polio virus vaccine is generally preferred, although the inactivated vaccine is still used in some countries (Holland, Sweden, Finland) and it is more appropriate in immunosuppressed individuals where a live vaccine might replicate with impunity. However, the live vaccine is cheaper, easier to administer, provides longer lasting immunity, and because it is administered orally it is able to elicit mucosal antibodies. However, a risk of reversion to a neurotrophic form is present, although this occurs very rarely – around two per million doses.

Rabies

The original vaccine against rabies was an attenuated virus produced by Louis Pasteur in the late 1800s by passaging between the brains of rabbits. The spinal cords of infected rabbits were then dried, which was found to reduce the virulence of the virus. However, many human vaccinees suffered from autoimmune paralytic disorders. The first inactivated vaccine was produced by Semple in 1911 by inactivation with phenol. Modern rabies vaccines are produced from virus propagated in human diploid cell lines and inactivated using β-propiolactone, although Semple-type vaccines remain in widespread use. Normally, inactivated rabies vaccine is given prophylactically to those at risk of bites from rabid animals (kennel workers, etc.) although it can be administered to bite victims *after* infection because of the comparatively slow migration of the virus from the site of the bite along the peripheral nerves to the brain.

Toxoids

Toxoids are inactivated bacterial toxins which provide acquired immunity to the toxin rather than to the bacterium itself. Examples include tetanus toxoid which is an inactivated toxin from *Clostridium tetani*, and diphtheria toxoid which is an inactivated toxin from *Corynebacterium diphtheriae.* Also in this category are vaccines made from the capsular polysaccharide of certain bacteria (Table 6.1).

Smallpox

The prototype of all live vaccines is against smallpox caused by variola virus. The history of smallpox and the development of the vaccines used to eliminate this disease are inextricably linked to the development of modern immunology. Until only recently, smallpox has been a significant cause of mortality throughout much of human history. It was known from ancient times that the disease only occurred once and survivors were then immune. This led to a common practice we now call **variolation** in which material was taken from the pocks on individuals with mild disease and used to infect children in the hope that the resultant disease would also be mild. In effect this was exploiting naturally occurring attenuated variola, although in practice this was an unpredictable and dangerous procedure. A safer practice was to infect with material from animal pocks. Although Edward Jenner is credited with conducting the first human trial with an experimental cowpox-derived vaccine in 1796, the observation that milkmaids who had caught cowpox were resistant to smallpox thereafter had been recognized much earlier. Vaccinia (named after the Latin *vacca* for cow) is also an animal pox virus which was used with great success in the 1960s and 1970s for the final elimination of smallpox. However, the origins of vaccinia are obscure, being more related to camelpox or horsepox than to cowpox (see Alcami and Smith, 1996).

Mycobacterium

The prototypic bacterial vaccine is BCG (Bacille Calmette–Guérin), which is an attenuated form of *M. bovis* that has been used as a prophylaxis for tuberculosis since the early 1920s. BCG is probably the most widely used vaccine, with over 3 billion vaccinations since it was first introduced. It has proved to be safe, with less than five fatalities per million. It can be given at any time from birth onwards, and a single dose can engender long-lasting immunity of anything from 5 to 50 years. However, its efficacy is limited; more can be learned about BCG in section 2.2.3.

6.2   Engineered vaccines

Despite spectacular successes in controlling some major human and animal infectious diseases, conventional vaccines have been made by trial and error, without any real understanding of the virulence of the pathogen or what constitutes an effective protective immune response. A better understanding of virulence and protective immunity should lead to a more rational and less empirical approach to the design of vaccines.

In the past decade a revolution in vaccine design has taken place, in which recombinant DNA technology ('genetic engineering') has been used to clone the genes encoding the microbial antigens (Figure 6.1). The gene, or the antigen it encodes, is then administered in a delivery vehicle according to the type of immune response desired. Four

Figure 6.1
Making vaccines using recombinant DNA technology.
Genes encoding the required antigens can be expressed as
recombinant proteins in bacteria or yeast and extracted, or
cloned in live attenuated vectors such as vaccinia virus or
BCG. Alternatively, synthetic peptides can be made according
to the encoded sequence. DNA itself can also be used by *in
vivo* transfection of tissues.

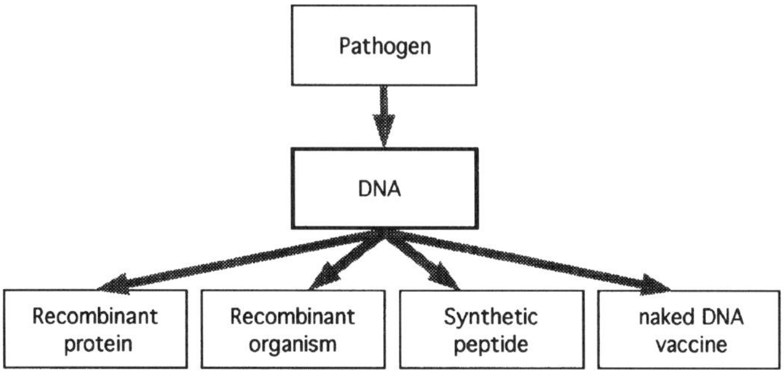

general strategies are being explored: **recombinant proteins,
synthetic peptides, live recombinant organisms** and **DNA
vaccines**. The successful design of an engineered vaccine is
strongly dependent on first knowing what kind of immune
response is protective and to which antigen of the pathogen
this protective response is directed. Added to these strategies
is a slightly different approach in which the gene(s) responsible for the virulence of a pathogen are knocked out using
genetic engineering. This is more complex as several genes
will normally account for the virulence of a pathogen; so far
only a few replication-defective viruses have been produced
(see Kit *et al.*, 1992; Beer *et al.*, 1997; Boursnell *et al.*, 1997).

There are several reasons why these new approaches to
vaccine design are attractive alternatives to more conventional means.

- First is the opportunity to design vaccines rationally. This
  concerns the antigenic composition of the vaccine itself
  as well as the particular delivery vehicle used and the
  type of immunity (antibodies and/or T_C cells) elicited.
- The second attraction is safety. Recombinant proteins
  and peptides are neither infectious nor pathogenic and
  obviate any concerns of reversion.
- A third advantage concerns the unlimited supply of
  antigen that can be made in host cells. This overcomes
  problems associated with making vaccines against microbes that are impossible to grow in culture.

6.2.1 *Recombinant proteins*

In order to obtain sufficiently large quantities of protein for vaccine production, rapidly dividing host cells are used. Bacteria are widely used, the most common being *Escherichia coli*, although if eukaryotic expression is desired, insect cells (using the baculovirus expression system) or yeast are also suitable as host cells. Recombinant proteins have the same immunological properties of inactivated conventional vaccines. That is, they require an adjuvant and booster immunizations, and although they elicit antibodies, they are poor inducers of T_C cells.

In recent years, novel adjuvants and delivery vehicles have been developed to increase the immunogenicity of exogenous antigens. Of note are the lipid delivery vehicles, such as liposomes and immune-stimulating complexes (ISCOMs), which can be used to elicit T_C-cell responses from recombinant proteins (see below).

Hepatitis B

Hepatitis B virus (HBV) is a major causative agent of liver cirrhosis and it is intimately associated with progression to hepatocellular carcinoma. During chronic infection the infected liver cells produce large quantities of S protein, a major component of the viral capsid. Far more is made than is needed for viral assembly and the excess is secreted into the blood where it self-assembles into 22-nm particles. These non-infectious particles became known as the **hepatitis B surface antigen** (HBsAg) because of their ability to elicit neutralizing antibodies in vaccinees. In practice, serum from carriers is first heated to inactivate any infectious HBV present, followed by screening for safety and efficacy in chimpanzees. However, this was an expensive procedure and yields are limited by the supply of human donors. The recombinant vaccine (McAleer *et al.*, 1984) consists of particles made in the yeast cells *Saccharomyces cerevisiae* (the particles were found not to assemble in *E. coli*) transformed with a plasmid expressing S gene. The particles are biochemically purified and administered with adjuvant (alum) by intramuscular injection as a prophylactic for healthcare workers and others exposed to human blood. This was the first, and currently the only, recombinant protein vaccine licenced for human use. New-generation recombinant vaccines that contain other envelope proteins (preS1 and preS2) are under development in the hope that they will be more immunogenic in people who do not respond well to S antigen alone (reviewed by Zuckerman, 1997).

Adjuvants/ISCOMs

Currently the most widely used adjuvant approved for human use is alum (aluminium hydroxide) although this is a relatively weak adjuvant that elicits only a mild inflammatory response. Several alternatives are being developed including the **liposome**, a lipid vesicle within which antigen is entrapped, and the **immune stimulating complex** or ISCOM (Mowat *et al.*, 1993). Both are made from lipids (usually phosphatidyl choline and cholesterol) although ISCOMs also incorporate saponin (a plant-derived glycoside surfactant used to solubilize proteins), which has strong adjuvant properties and which seems to confer ISCOMs with the ability to induce higher titres of antibodies than other adjuvants. Importantly, these lipid delivery vehicles are also able to elicit CD8+ T_C-cell responses to soluble antigen that would otherwise only elicit antibody. Lipid carriers fuse with the plasma membrane of antigen-presenting cells thereby delivering the antigen directly into the cytosol and into the HLA class I antigen-processing pathway (see Figure 1.3).

Another useful adjuvant for inducing mucosal immunity to antigens is cholera toxin derived from the enteric bacterium *Vibrio cholerae* (see section 2.1.1). The non-toxic B-subunit can be conjugated to orally administered antigens, which targets them to the intestinal mucosa and acts as a strong adjuvant leading to the production of secretory IgA (Holmgren *et al.*, 1993). It also overcomes the natural tendency of protein antigens administered across mucosal membranes to elicit antigen-specific hyporesponsiveness (or **mucosal tolerance**).

6.2.2 *Synthetic peptides*

Epitopes recognized by T and B lymphocytes can often be mimicked by peptides. These can be deduced from the nucleotide sequence of a gene using the genetic code. Peptides can then be produced chemically by sequentially coupling amino acids together in a peptide synthesizer. The epitope bound by immunoglobulin consists of a footprint on the surface of the antigen and occasionally may comprise amino acids that are contiguous in the primary amino acid sequence. These linear B-cell epitopes can be mimicked by synthetic peptides, and can often be used to elicit antibodies that will cross-react with the native antigen. In most cases, however, the amino acids involved in B-cell epitopes are scattered throughout the primary sequence and are only juxtaposed when the antigen is folded into its native conformation. These topographic epitopes are not easily mimicked by synthetic peptides. In contrast, T-cell epitopes are always linear, contiguous sequences, and are therefore readily mimicked by synthetic peptides.

In every case, the choice of which particular peptide sequence to use as a vaccine is dependent on the prior mapping of dominant epitopes within the antigen that are recognized by protective antibodies or T cells. If neutralizing antibodies or protective T cells can be obtained from immune individuals, epitope mapping can be achieved by testing panels of synthetic peptides (**pepscanning**) for recognition in appropriate B- and T-cell assays (see Van der Zee *et al.*, 1989; Wang *et al.*, 1990; Kast *et al.*, 1991).

Alternatively, means are available to predict where linear T and B epitopes are located using only the primary amino acid sequence of the antigen. B-cell epitopes are surface-located and therefore composed mainly of hydrophilic residues. By scanning the primary amino acid sequence of a protein for stretches of hydrophilic regions it is possible to identify putative linear B-cell epitopes (see Hopp and Woods, 1981). In contrast, T-cell epitopes consist of residues with hydrophobic and hydrophilic side chains; the former generally point down into the peptide-binding cleft of the MHC molecule, whereas the latter generally point upwards towards the TCR. A useful predictive algorithm, particularly for class I MHC-presented epitopes, depends on the possession of so-called **anchor residues** which determine the specificity of peptide binding for particular allelic variants of MHC molecules (Rammensee *et al.*, 1993; Rotzschke and Falk, 1994). These motifs can be used to locate putative MHC-binding peptides within primary amino acid sequences (see Hill *et al.*, 1992).

The induction of antibodies by peptides usually requires the incorporation of a source of helper T-cell epitopes because B-cell epitopes alone are unable to engender antibodies. This can be achieved by synthesizing a peptide that incorporates both T_H- and B-cell epitopes, or by coupling the B cell to a large carrier protein. It is important to stress at this point that if immunological memory is desired from the peptide vaccine, the helper epitopes or the carrier protein must also be derived from the same pathogen as the B-cell epitopes. Peptides of T-cell epitopes can make excellent vaccines in inbred animal models, particularly against viral infections (reviewed by Melief and Kast, 1995). These are thought to be able to bypass antigen processing and bind directly to MHC molecules on antigen-presenting cells. The major hurdle for using peptides in humans, however, concerns their HLA-restricted presentation. In human populations, in which there is extensive MHC polymorphism, different epitopes must be identified for each of the most abundant HLA alleles. There are also conflicting data concerning whether helper T-cell epitopes are needed for the induction of T_C cells. Many studies have shown that T_C-cell epitopes can often be used for vaccination purposes without modification. It is possible that at sufficiently high peptide concentrations the need for helper determinants is overcome.

6.2.3 *Live recombinant organisms*

Using genetic engineering, attenuated pathogens can be used as vectors for foreign genes encoding the antigens of other pathogens. Upon immunization, the recombinant organism expresses both its own genes and the foreign gene(s) which provides antigen for acquired immunity. Most of the research effort has been used making recombinants of established attenuated vaccine strains such as vaccinia and BCG. Others such as adenovirus and herpes simplex virus, and intracellular bacteria such as *Salmonella*, are also being developed (Table 6.2). Each vector is being developed to exploit particular features of its infection. Viruses are particularly useful for eliciting T_C-cell responses to foreign antigens, whereas enteric organisms such as *Salmonella* are useful for eliciting mucosal immunity. Like the attenuated

Table 6.2 Examples of recombinant organisms as potential vaccines in humans

Lactococcus, Streptococcus, Escherichia	Commensal bacteria that could be used for mucosal delivery of foreign antigens and production of mucosal immunity, secretory IgA
Salmonella	Intracellular bacterium that induces T_C cells and antibodies; administered orally so also induces secretory IgA
Vaccinia virus	Animal pox virus administered by scarification of skin; infects many cell types and induces good T_C-cell responses; attenuated vaccinia and avipox viruses under development
Picornaviruses (poliovirus, rhinovirus)	Chimeric capsid VP1 and VP2 proteins have been engineered to contain short peptide sequences; administered nasally or orally so will induce secretory IgA
Adenovirus	Replication deficient mutants generated by gene knockout; used for the delivery of antigenic or therapeutic transgenes to cells *ex vivo* and *in vivo*
Herpes simplex virus	Replication deficient mutants generated by gene knockout; elicit antibodies and T_C cells; useful for gene delivery to nerve cells

Figure 6.2
Production of a recombinant virus using a transfer vector.
A cassette containing the foreign gene and regulatory sequences (promoter and
polyadenylation signals) is inserted into a copy of the target viral gene held within a transfer
vector. The resulting recombinant is transfected into cells which are co-infected with wild-
type virus. The transgene and regulatory sequences are inserted into the viral genome by
homologous recombination.

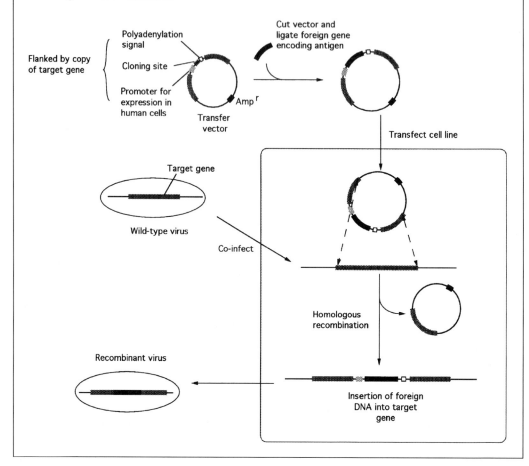

parental vaccine strains the recombinant should not require
adjuvants and the immunity engendered should be long
lasting.

In order to produce stable recombinants, the foreign gene
is usually integrated into a target gene within the genome
of the host organism using a process called **homologous
recombination**. Because the genomes of these organisms are
often too large for direct manipulation, the foreign gene is
usually first cloned into a smaller **transfer vector** derived
from a bacterial plasmid. A generalized strategy is depicted
in Figure 6.2. In the transfer vector is a copy of the target

gene of the intended host organism, into which the foreign gene is inserted. The recombinant transfer vector is then introduced into the host bacterium or, in the case of viruses, a cell infected with wild-type virus, which allows recombination between the shared sequences in the transfer vector and the target gene.

Pox viruses

Vaccinia was the first virus to be engineered as a vector for the expression of heterologous genes (reviewed by Carroll and Moss, 1997) and has been used to protect experimental animals against a multitude of diseases including those caused by influenza virus, hepatitis B virus, rabies virus, measles virus, and many others (see examples in Moss *et al.*, 1984; Wiktor *et al.*, 1984; Cremer *et al.*, 1985; Smith *et al.*, 1986; Drillen *et al.*, 1988).

Because of the large genome (> 180 kb), vaccinia can accommodate large amounts of foreign DNA, although a transfer vector is necessary. A vaccinia transfer vector is based on a bacterial plasmid containing an origin of replication for propagation in *E. coli* and the ampicillin resistance gene for selection of transformed bacteria. The site of insertion into vaccinia is usually made into a gene that is non-essential for replication, such as the thymidine kinase (*tk*) gene. This is achieved by cloning the foreign transgene and its necessary regulatory sequences into a vaccinia *tk* gene held in the transfer vector (Figure 6.2). This construct is then transfected into a suitable mammalian cell line, which is co-infected with wild-type vaccinia virus to allow homologous recombination to occur. Recombination causes inactivation of the *tk* gene, which confers resistance to the toxic thymidine analogue bromodeoxyuridine (BrdU). This can be used to select recombinant viruses from unwanted non-recombinants during the subsequent cloning and expansion steps.

Despite the potential of recombinant vaccinia virus there are risks associated with its use. A serious complication is vaccinia gangrene, in which the pock caused at the site of inoculation fails to heal. This occurs almost exclusively in patients who are immunosuppressed. A rarer but potentially fatal complication is viral encephalomyelitis (infection in the brain). Less serious complications include transmission to other sites such as the eye, systemic viraemia, and allergic reactions. Although these effects are seldom seen in healthy people, several safer pox viruses are being developed as alternatives to vaccinia. These include NYVAC, which

has been derived from vaccinia by the deletion of 18 open
reading frames. NYVAC has a much reduced virulence and
a far more limited host range. Another highly attenuated
vaccinia virus is modified virus Ankara (MVA), a replication deficient strain that was developed towards the end of
the smallpox eradication campaign (Carroll *et al.*, 1997). Finally, several members of the family avipoxviridae, including fowlpox and canarypox, are being developed as vectors.
These viruses have a restricted tropism for avian cells and,
although they will infect mammalian cells, they are unable
to replicate (Carroll and Moss, 1997).

Adenoviruses

Disabled adenoviruses are highly efficient vectors for the
transfer of heterologous genes to human cells both *in vivo*
and *in vitro*. These are used mainly for gene therapy applications, but also have potential for vaccination (see reviews
by Mitani and Caskey, 1993; Imler, 1995). Adenoviruses types
4, 5 and 7 are usually used because of their ability to infect
humans without causing disease. The E1 gene encodes a
transactivation factor that is required for the expression of
other early and late genes, and so plays a pivotal role in
viral replication. The first disabled adenoviruses were made
lacking the E1 gene in order to block viral replication. These
mutant viruses can only be propagated in a 'helper' cell line
that constitutively expresses the E1 protein, which substi-
tutes for the defect in the E1 deletion mutant (Figure 6.3).
The progeny viruses that are released from the helper cell
line are infective but are replication defective owing to the
E1 deletion. Second-generation vectors with additional dele-
tions in E2 and E4 to reduce background gene expression
are also being tested. In the context of vaccines, recombinant disabled adenoviruses can be made by inserting foreign
transgenes either before transfection or by using homologous recombination as shown in Figure 6.3. E3 is also usually
deleted to ensure that the class I MHC-processing pathway
is not inhibited by E3/19K in infected host cells (see section 3.2). Replication-defective adenoviruses are particularly useful for the delivery of immunogenic or therapeutic
transgenes because there is little or no background expression of endogenous viral genes. Moreover, using appropriate
promoters, the levels of expression of the transgene can be
very high.

Adenoviruses have a natural tropism for oropharyngeal
and respiratory epithelium and experimental adenovirus-
based vaccines expressing transgenes are usually administered

Figure 6.3
Construction of a recombinant adenovirus.
An adenovirus vector is made from wild-type virus by deleting
the E1 gene responsible for transactivation of other viral genes.
Recombinant viruses are made by transfecting the mutated
adenovirus genome into the 293 helper cell line which
constitutively expresses E1, and cotransfecting with a transfer
plasmid as described in Figure 6.2. E1 supplied by the helper
cell transactivates viral genes and allows the E1 defective
viruses to replicate. The progeny remain disabled and although
able to infect human cells will be unable to replicate (unless
co-infected by wild-type adenovirus able to supply the helper
functions).

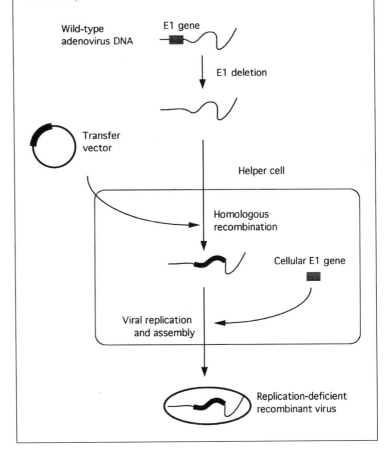

orally in animal models. By this route the vaccines are useful for eliciting specific mucosal immunity to the transgene
product. Because the vaccine is live, long-lasting immunity
is achieved from just a single inoculation, and consists of
both T_C cells and antibody-mediated immune responses.
Thus these vectors have the potential for the development
of vaccines to other mucosal pathogens.

Chimeric virus capsids

A slight variation on this theme is the engineering of viral capsid proteins to contain heterologous sequences of amino acids, ranging from short peptide epitopes to whole antigens. This has been achieved with polio virus and rhinovirus (both picornaviridae) which have been engineered to contain short peptide sequences corresponding to linear B- and T-cell epitopes (Evans and Almond, 1991; Arnold *et al.*, 1996). However, only relatively short peptides can be inserted, as sequences longer that 15 or so amino acids interfere with capsid assembly. Longer sequences can be attached to the termini of the major capsid protein of papillomavirus which self-assembles *in vitro* (see Lowy, 1994); it is likely these fusion particles can be used to elicit both antibodies and T_C cells. In addition to vaccine design, the modification of viral capsids and envelope proteins will also have useful applications in gene therapy for the delivery of therapeutic transgenes in viruses to novel target cells (reviewed by Harris and Lemoine, 1996).

Recombinant bacteria

A number of bacteria are also being developed as live recombinant vaccines (Table 6.2). Because of their larger genomes, bacteria have the potential to carry more foreign DNA than most viruses. These species under study include the intracellular bacteria *Mycobacterium bovis* Bacille Calmette–Guérin (BCG), *Salmonella typhimurium* and *Listeria monocytogenes* (see reviews by Stover *et al.*, 1991; Flynn, 1994; Cirillo *et al.*, 1995; Jensen *et al.*, 1997a, b). Commensal bacteria such as *Streptococcus gordonii* are also being developed as vectors for the delivery of antigens to the intestinal tract.

In humans, the BCG vaccine is normally administered intradermally and has been found to elicit strong cell-mediated (T_C-cell and DTH responses) as well as antibodymediated immunity. In animals, orally or nasally administered BCG engenders T_C cells and DTH in the intestines, respiratory epithelium and other mucosal sites, as well as secretory IgA and serum IgG (Stover *et al.*, 1991). It is hoped that recombinant BCG can be used for the development of vaccines against other pathogens that gain entry across mucosal membranes, such as HIV, genital HPVs and herpes simplex virus.

Salmonella and *Listeria* are also intracellular bacteria that have been transformed with plasmids that express foreign antigens (Table 6.2). *Salmonella typhimurium* has a tropism for intestinal epithelium and persists for long periods after oral immunization by penetrating intestinal macrophages. Attenuated strains of *Salmonella* are attractive live vaccine candidates because they have been found to be immunogenic by nasal, oral, vaginal and rectal routes of entry, wherein they elicit strong mucosal and systemic T_C-cell and antibody responses. *Listeria monocytogenes* is also an intracellular bacterium that enters the cytoplasm of infected cells and is a potent stimulator of T_C-cell responses. The human commensal *Streptococcus gordonii* has also been used as a means for delivering foreign antigens to the mucosa and stimulating the production of antigen-specific secretory IgA and serum IgG. As with recombinant BCG, it is hoped that these vaccines can be used to protect against other pathogens that gain entry across the anogenital and intestinal mucosae.

6.2.4 *Nucleic acid vaccines*

The efficient delivery of transgenes into cells *in vivo* is best accomplished using virus vectors such as adenoviruses or retroviruses. Naked DNA, in contrast, is taken up by cells much less efficiently. Yet despite this, naked DNA is a very effective means of eliciting immune responses to the encoded antigens (Waine and McManus, 1995; Ulmer *et al.*, 1996; Donnelly *et al.*, 1997). There is now tremendous interest in DNA vaccines, in part because the simplicity with which DNA vaccines can be made may obviate the need to make and purify recombinant proteins and organisms, and the versatility that this technology has to offer.

The majority of currently used DNA vaccines are constructed according to the same basic design. They are based on bacterial plasmids to allow their propagation in *E. coli*, and contain the gene encoding the antigen located downstream of a promoter that is operational in human cells. The promoter of choice is the intermediate–early promoter of human cytomegalovirus (CMV), although other promoters have been used. Many vaccines also employ an intron between the promoter and the antigen coding sequence, which is reported to give better levels of gene expression. In animals, the administration of DNA can be by several different routes, but the intramuscular and intradermal routes are most commonly used in experimental animals. A device called a gene gun has been developed for intradermal immunization that propels DNA-coated, 1–3 µm, gold particles into the skin (Fynan *et al.*, 1993). This appears to transfect cells more efficiently than intramuscular injection because smaller amounts of DNA are required to achieve immunization. The relative merits of these and other routes (such as intranasal and scarification into the skin) are still under scrutiny, but in general, better T_H1-type responses are elicited by intramuscular injection, whereas T_H2-type responses are preferentially induced by the gene gun.

The relative ease with which genomic expression libraries can be constructed from pathogens has meant that whole genomes can be used to immunize (Barry et al., 1995). In practice, expression library immunization (ELI) is being used as a means for screening whole genomes to discover the appropriate antigens to include into subunit vaccines, rather than as a vaccine in itself.

An important and useful property of DNA vaccines is their ability to elicit both cytotoxic and humoral immune responses. For example, in the first study of this kind (Ulmer et al., 1993), the delivery of the nucleoprotein (NP) gene of influenza virus into mice by intramuscular injection elicited NP-specific antibodies and T_C cells. Moreover, these animals were protected against a challenge of live influenza virus. Many subsequent studies in animals have shown that protective immunity can be engendered to a variety of live pathogens (see, for example, Sedegah et al., 1994; Xiang et al., 1994; Donnelly et al., 1996).

There are many unanswered questions about DNA vaccines, not least of which concern the site of antigen production and presentation to the immune system. Skin contains an abundance of professional antigen-presenting cells (APCs) including tissue macrophages and Langerhans cells (cutaneous dendritic cells) which may become directly transfected during intradermal immunization. Dendritic cells migrate back to draining lymph nodes where presentation of antigen to naive T cells occurs. In intramuscular administration, muscle cells become transfected and become the site in which the antigen is produced. However, muscle cells do not normally possess the costimulatory molecules required for the activation of naive T lymphocytes. Therefore the antigen is probably acquired in some way by professional APCs within the muscle, which then migrate to draining lymph nodes. Alternatively, soluble antigen may be carried back to the lymph nodes in draining lymph fluid where it may be picked up by professional APCs. Recent studies have shown that prokaryotic DNA itself has stimulatory properties and is able to activate professional APCs to release the T_H1-inducing cytokines IL-12 and IFN-γ. Indeed, specific sequences of non-methylated non-mammalian DNA have been identified that act as powerful adjuvants for T_H1-mediated immunity (Klinman *et al.*, 1996). Less is known about how to manipulate DNA vaccines to generate stronger T_H2-type responses, although incorporating appropriate T_H2-type cytokines may help (Xiang and Ertl, 1995).

There are also safety issues that need to be addressed before DNA vaccines can be used safely in humans. The main one is the slight chance of random integration of the DNA into the genome of cells transfected *in vivo*. This may lead to the interruption of important cellular genes (**insertional mutagenesis**) which may predispose the cell to becoming a cancer cell. In practice, the frequency of random recombination is vanishingly small (Nichols *et al.*, 1995) and no more frequent than integration of DNA from commensal microorganisms. Another concern stems from the persistence of DNA, which may remain active for months after immunization. This may lead to chronic exposure to the immune system of antigen leading either to tolerance of the antigen or autoimmunity.

Summary

- Vaccines against pathogens are conventionally made by inactivation or attenuation of the organism such that it is no longer pathogenic whilst retaining its immunogenicity. Most conventional vaccines are designed to engender prophylactic immunity based on neutralizing antibodies. Most are against viruses, there are fewer vaccines available for bacteria, and there are none against parasites. A number of bacterial (subunit) vaccines have been derived from polysaccharide capsules, although these elicit weak T-cell immunity and memory. Inactivated pathogens require adjuvants to be immunogenic, the immunity elicited after immunization is relatively short term, and booster immunizations are required to maintain sufficiently high levels of antibodies. In contrast, attenuated organisms tend to elicit longer-lasting immunity (sometimes for life) without adjuvants and with a single immunization. Moreover, attenuated viruses and intracellular bacteria retain their ability to elicit T_C cells as well as antibodies. However, live attenuated organisms have the potential to revert and become pathogenic.

- Recombinant DNA technology promises to overcome some of the problems associated with conventional approaches, such as safety and short supply. It will also allow vaccines to new pathogens to be developed, for existing vaccines to be improved, and for vaccines to cancer, autoimmunity and other diseases to be designed rationally. Subunit vaccines can be made by expressing antigens from their genes in bacteria or yeast, or by deducing the encoded amino acid sequence and producing synthetic peptides. Novel delivery systems provide the opportunity to elicit T_C cells and develop therapeutic subunit vaccines. Another approach is to engineer attenuated organisms to express the foreign antigens, thereby vastly enhancing their immunogenicity. In recent years, genetic immunization ('DNA vaccines') has appeared, which promises to make the tasks of producing engineered vaccines and screening for relevant antigens much simpler. Attenuation may also be achieved by DNA manipulation; so far only replication-deficient viruses have been made. The virulence of bacteria and parasites is multigenic so will require multiple gene knockouts to render the organism safe.

Study problems

1. What is the difference between attenuated and inactivated vaccines, and what are the good and bad features associated with them?
2. How in principle are recombinant adenoviruses and vaccinia viruses made?
3. What are the relative merits of using recombinant vaccinia and adenoviruses and how may the problems (if any) be overcome?
4. How might a recombinant protein be used to elicit (a) T_C cells and (b) antibodies?
5. What are the pros and cons of synthetic peptide vaccines (hint: think of T_C-cell responses *and* antibody responses)?
6. How are nucleic acid vaccines thought to work?

Selected reading

Alcami, A. and Smith, G.L., 1996, Receptors for gamma-interferon encoded by poxviruses: implications for the unknown origin of vaccinia virus, *Trends Microbiol.*, **4**, 321–326

Arnold, G.F., Resnick, D.A., Smith, A.D., Geisler, S.C., Holmes, A.K. and Arnold, E., 1996, Chimeric rhinoviruses as tools for vaccine development and characterization of protein epitopes, *Intervirology*, **39**, 72–78

Barry, M.A., Lai, W.C. and Johnston, S.A., 1995, Protection against mycoplasma-infection using expression-library immunization, *Nature*, **377**, 632–635

Beer, B., Baier, M., zur Megede, J., Norley, S. and Kurth, R., 1997, Vaccine effect using a live attenuated *nef*-deficient simian immunodeficiency virus of African green monkeys in the absence of detectable vaccine virus replication *in vivo*, *Proc. Natl. Acad. Sci. USA*, **94**, 4062–4067

Boursnell, M.E.G., Entwisle, C., Blakeley, D., Roberts, C., Duncan, I.A., Chisholm, S.E., Martin, G.M., Jennings, R., Challanain, D.N., Sobek, I., Inglis, S.C. and McLean, C.S., 1997, Genetically inactivated herpes simplex virus type 2 (HSV-2) vaccine provides effective protection against primary and recurrent HSV-2 disease, *J. Infect. Dis.*, **175**, 16–25

Carroll, M.W. and Moss, B., 1997, Poxviruses as expression vectors, *Curr. Opin. Biotech.*, **8**, 573–577

Carroll, M.W., Overwijk, W.W., Chamberlain, R.S., Rosenberg, S.A., Moss, B. and Restifo, N.P., 1997, Highly attenuated modified vaccinia virus Ankara (MVA) as an effective recombinant vector: a murine tumor model, *Vaccine*, **15**, 387–394

Cirillo, J.D., Stover, C.K., Bloom, B.R., Jacobs, W.R. and Barletta, R.G., 1995, Bacterial vaccine vectors and Bacille Calmette–Guérin, *Clin. Infect. Dis.*, **20**, 1001–1009

Cremer, K., Mackett, M., Wohlenberg, C., Notkins, A.L. and Moss, B., 1985, Vaccinia virus recombinants expressing herpes simplex virus type 1 glycoprotein D prevent latent herpes in mice, *Science*, **228**, 737–740

Donnelly, J.J., Martinez, D., Jansen, K.U., Ellis, R.W., Montgomery, D.L. and Liu, M.A., 1996, Protection against papillomavirus with a polynucleotide vaccine, *J. Infect. Dis.*, **173**, 314–320

Donnelly, J.J., Ullmer, J.B., Shiver, J.W. and Lin, M.A., 1997, DNA vaccines, *Annu. Rev. Immunol.*, **15**, 617–648

Drillen, R., Sphener, D., Kirn, A., Giraudon, P., Buckland, R., Wild, F. and Lecocq, J.-P., 1988, Protection of mice from fatal measles encephalitis by vacciniation with vaccinia virus recombinants encoding either the haemagglutinin or the fusion protein, *Proc. Natl. Acad. Sci. USA*, **85**, 1252–1256

Evans, D.J. and Almond, J.W., 1991, Design, construction, and characterization of poliovirus antigen chimeras, *Meth. Enzymol.*, **203**, 86–400

Flynn, J.L., 1994, Recombinant BCG as an antigen delivery system, *Cell. Molec. Biol.*, **40**, 31–36

Fynan, E.F., Webster, R.G., Fuller, D.H., Haynes, J.R., Santoro, J.C. and Robinson, H.L., 1993, DNA vaccines – protective immunizations by parenteral, mucosal, and gene-gun inoculations, *Proc. Natl. Acad. Sci. USA*, **90**, 11 478–11 482

Harris, J.D. and Lemoine, N.R., 1996, Strategies for targeted gene therapy, *Trends Genet.*, **12**, 400–405

Hill, A.V.S., Elvin, J., Willis, A.C., Aidoo, M., Allsopp, C.E.M., Gotch, F.M., Gao, X.M., Takiguchi, M., Greenwood, B.M., Townsend, A.R.M., McMichael, A.J. and Whittle, H.C., 1992, Molecular analysis of the association of HLA-B 53 and resistance to severe malaria, *Nature*, **360**, 434–439

Holmgren, J., Lycke, N. and Czerkinsky, C., 1993, Cholera-toxin and cholera-B subunit as oral mucosal adjuvant and antigen vector systems, *Vaccine*, **11**, 1179–1184

Hopp, T.P. and Woods, K.R., 1981, Prediction of protein antigenic determinants from amino-acid sequences, *Proc. Natl. Acad. Sci. USA*, **78**, 3824–3828

Imler, J.L., 1995, Adenovirus vectors as recombinant viral vaccines, *Vaccine*, **13**, 1143–1151

Jensen, E.R., Selvakumar, R., Shen, H., Ahmed, R., Wettstein, F.O. and Miller, J.F., 1997a, Recombinant *Listeria monocytogenes* vacciniation eliminates papillomavirus-induced tumours and prevents papilloma formation from viral DNA, *J. Virol.*, **71**, 8467–8474

Jensen, E.R., Shen, H., Wettstein, F.O., Ahmed, R. and Miller, J.F., 1997b, Recombinant *Listeria monocytogenes* as a live vaccine vehicle and a probe for studying cell-mediated immunity, *Immunol. Rev.*, **158**, 147–157

Kast, W.M., Roux, L., Curren, J., Blom, H.J.J., Voordouw, A.C., Meloen, R.H., Kolakofsky, D., Melief, C.J.M., 1991, Protection against lethal sendai virus-infection by *in vivo* priming of virus-specific cytotoxic lymphocytes-T with a free synthetic peptide, *Proc. Natl. Acad. Sci. USA*, **88**, 2283–2287

Kit, S., Otsuka, H. and Kit, M., 1992, Expression of porcine pseudorabies virus genes by a bovine herpesvirus-1 (infectious bovine-rhinotracheitis virus) vector, *Arch. Virol.*, **124**, 1–20

Klinman, D.M., Yi, A.K., Beaucage, S.L., Conover, J. and Krieg, A.M., 1996, CpG motifs present in bacterial-DNA rapidly induce lymphocytes to secrete interleukin-6, interleukin-12, and interferon-gamma, *Proc. Natl. Acad. Sci. USA*, **93**, 2879–2883

Lowy, D.R., 1994, Genital human papillomavirus infection, *Proc. Natl. Acad. Sci. USA*, **91**, 2436–2440

McAleer, W.J., Buynak, E.B., Maigetter, R.Z., Wampler, D.E., Miller, W.J. and Hilleman, M.R., 1984, Human hepatitis B vaccine from recombinant yeast, *Nature*, **307**, 178–180

Melief, C.J.M. and Kast, W.M., 1995, T-cell immunotherapy of tumors by adoptive transfer of cytotoxic T lymphocytes and by vaccination with minimal essential epitopes, *Immunol. Rev.*, **145**, 167–177

Mitani, K. and Caskey, C.T., 1993, Delivering therapeutic genes – matching approach and application, *Trends Biotechnol.*, **11**, 162–166

Moss, B., Smith, G.L., Gerin, J.L. and Purcell, R.H., 1984, Live recombinant vaccinia virus protects chimpanzees against hepatitis B, *Nature*, **311**, 67–69

Mowat, A.M., Maloy, K.J. and Donachie, A.M., 1993, Immune stimulating complexes as adjuvants for inducing local and systemic immunity after oral immunization with protein antigens, *Immunology*, **80**, 527–534

Nichols, W.W., Ledwith, B.J., Manam, S.V. and Troilo, P.J., 1995, Potential DNA vaccine integration into host-cell genome, *Ann. N.Y. Acad. Sci.*, **772**, 30–39

Rammensee, H.G., Falk, K. and Rotzschke, O., 1993, Peptides naturally presented by MHC class-I molecules, *Annu. Rev. Immunol.*, **11**, 213–244

Rotzschke, O. and Falk, K., 1994, Origin, structure and motifs of naturally processed MHC class-II ligands, *Curr. Opin. Immunol.*, **6**, 45–51

Sedegah, M., Hedstrom, R., Hobart, P. and Hoffman, S.L., 1994, Protection against malaria by immunization with plasmid DNA encoding circumsporozoite protein, *Proc. Natl. Acad. Sci. USA*, **91**, 9866–9870

Smith, G.L., Murphy, B.R. and Moss, B., 1986, Construction and characterization of an infectious vaccinia virus recombinant that expresses influenza virus haemagglutinin and induces resistance to influenza virus infection in hamsters, *Proc. Natl. Acad. Sci. USA*, **80**, 7155–7159

Stover, C.K., Delacruz, V.F., Fuerst, T.R., Burlein, J.E., Benson, L.A., Bennett, L.T., Bansal, G.P., Young, J.F., Lee, M.H., Hatfull, G.F., Snapper, S.B., Barletta, R.G., Jacobs, W.R. and Bloom, B.R., 1991, New use of BCG for recombinant vaccines, *Nature*, **351**, 456–460

Ulmer, J.B., Donnelly, J.J., Parker, S.E., Rhodes, G.H., Felgner, P.L., Dwarki, V.J., Gromkowski, S.H., Deck, R.R., Dewitt, C.M., Friedman, A., Hawe, L.A., Leandor, K.R., Martinez, D., Perry, H.C., Shiver, J.W., Montgomery, D.L. and Liu, M.A., 1993, Heterologous protection against influenza by injection of DNA encoding a viral protein, *Science*, **259**, 1745–1749

Ulmer, J.B., Sadoff, J.C. and Liu, M.A., 1996, DNA vaccines, *Curr. Opin. Immunol.*, **8**, 531–536

Van der Zee, R., Vaneden, W., Meloen, R.H., Noordzij, A. and Van Embden, J.D.A., 1989, Efficient mapping and characterization of a T-cell epitope by the simultaneous synthesis of multiple peptides, *Eur. J. Immunol.*, **19**, 43–47

Waine, G.J. and McManus, D.P., 1995, Nucleic acids: vaccines of the future, *Parasitol. Today*, **11**, 113–116

Wang, J.-G., Jansen, R.W., Brown, E.A. and Lemon, S.M., 1990, Immunogenic domains of hepatitis delta-virus antigen-peptide-mapping of epitopes recognized by human and woodchuck antibodies, *J. Virol.*, **64**, 1108–1116

Wiktor, T.J., MacFarlan, R.I., Reagan, K.J., Dietzschold, B., Curtis, P.J., Wunner, W.H., Kieny, M.P., Lathe, R., Lecocq, J.P., Mackett, M., Moss, B. and Koprowski, H., 1984, Protection from rabies by a vaccinia virus recombinant containing the rabies virus glycoprotein gene, *Proc. Natl. Acad. Sci. USA*, **81**, 7194–7198

Xiang, Z.Q. and Ertl, H.C., 1995, Manipulation of the immune response to a plasmid-encoded viral antigen by coinoculation with a plasmid expressing cytokines, *Immunity*, **2**, 129–135

Xiang, Z.Q., Spitalnik, S., Tran, M., Wunner, W.H., Cheng, J. and Ertl, H.C., 1994, Vaccination against the rabies virus glycoprotein gene induces protective immunity against rabies virus, *Virology*, **199**, 132–140

Zuckerman, J., 1997, Vaccination against viral hepatitis, *Curr. Opin. Infect. Dis.*, **10**, 379–384

Index